THE CONQUEST OF SMALLPOX:

The Impact of Inoculation on Smallpox Mortality in Eighteenth Century Britain

Peter Razzell

Caliban Books

© Peter Razzell 1977

First published 1977 by
CALIBAN BOOKS
13 The Dock, Firle, Sussex BN8 6NY
(*Telephone* Glynde 335)

ISBN 0 904573 03 6

To the memory of my mother and father

CONTENTS

PREFACE

In a recent edition of the *Lancet*, Professor McKeown's thesis that "medical intervention has made a relatively small contribution to the prevention of sickness and death" has been discussed as a serious part of a policy debate on the allocation of resources between conventional and environmental medicine. Dr Lever, commenting on this claim, has accepted that "improvements in nutrition and hygiene and changes in behaviour can take most of the credit" for decreasing mortality, and that the publicity in favour of environmental medicine coming out of McKeown's work, "is of a type likely to affect Ministers."[1] The present book can be seen in part as an attempt to show that historically, one classical conventional phophylactic measure—inoculation against smallpox (variolation)—was dramatically effective in reducing overall mortality.

At a general level, the case for the role of prophylactic measures against smallpox can be demonstrated quite unambiguously. During the first seven years after the introduction of civil registration (1838-44), only about one-and-a-half per cent of children born in England and Wales died of smallpox, in spite of it being a universal disease of young children—87 per cent of all deaths occurred under the age of ten—with a case-fatality rate of approximately forty per cent. Given that we know that smallpox is a disease which potentially attacks everyone at all ages (except for a small minority of about five per cent with natural immunity), and that it was a universal disease affecting nearly everybody before the medical introduction of variolation in 1721, this represents a very dramatic saving of life. In the absence of variolation and vaccination, between one in four and one in three more children born would have died than actually did in early Victorian England, and this figure takes no account of the effects of secondary diseases. It is probable that the more serious of these, such as broncho-pneumonia—and there is evidence to show that this complication affected most of the more severe cases of smallpox—significantly increased overall mortality from smallpox before it was brought under control.

The main perspective from which the present book was written was a demographic one, and recent research in India has yielded findings of particular significance to this perspective. It has been established that smallpox is one of the major causes of male infertility, through the creation of focal lesions in the epidydimis. There is some historical evidence that smallpox in Britain had a significant effect on fertility, and that with the disappearance of the disease fertility increased. Although it is impossible to put a precise figure to the combined effect of decreasing mortality and increasing fertility, it is clear that the gradual elimination of smallpox was of profound demographic importance. Its conquest was achieved through inoculation and vaccination; the former was a product of folk medicine, the latter an unintended and accidental attenuation of this inoculation. Smallpox ranks with bubonic plague in its historical importance, and without its gradual elimination, the world's population would have suffered the kind of decimation resulting from the Black Death, and the Industrial Revolution of the late eighteenth and the early nineteenth century would not have been possible.

One of the lessons to emerge from this book, is that effective medical measures do not always come from highly organized and expensive research programmes, but sometimes arise out of the traditional skills of folk medicine—the wisdom of the ordinary man. (Perhaps more money should be spent on the evaluation of the effectiveness of all forms of folk medicine). The conquest of smallpox was undoubtedly the greatest achievement in the history of medicine—with the exception perhaps of malaria and yellow fever, the prevention or cure of no other disease remotely resembles the importance of smallpox prophylaxsis— and the numerous nameless inoculators and vaccinators practising during the past two hundred and fifty years and more, are the true heroes of this book.

INTRODUCTION

In 1803 a correspondent wrote to the *Gentleman's Magazine* about the late eighteenth century population increase in England:

> "One very great cause of increasing population may be ascribed to the success of inoculation for smallpox. One in four or five, or about 200 to 250 in a thousand, usually died of this loathsome disorder in the natural way of infection . . . so that this saving of lives alone would account for our increasing number, without perplexing ourselves for any other causes."[2]

Such a sweeping claim invites scepticism, but recent work in historical demography suggests that we should take it more seriously than medical historians have hitherto. T. H. Hollingsworth, in his definitive work on the demography of the British peerage, concluded that there was a marked increase in expectation of life during the middle of the eighteenth century, which is the period when inoculation became widespread amongst the aristocracy. This change may be summarized by the following Table on the mortality experiences of aristocratic women[3]:

Cohort Born	Expectation of life at birth (years)
1700-24	36.3
1725-49	36.7
1750-74	45.7
1775-99	49.0
1800-24	51.7

Almost identical results emerged from a study I made of gentry families living in the counties of Northamptonshire and Hertfordshire, but with an even larger increase in life-expectancy: from 35 years in 1720-39 to 48 years in 1740-59.[4] Data from the study of life annuities and tontines for the same period lead to an almost identical conclusion,[5] and it must now be considered to be a firm finding, at least for aristocratic and gentry groups.

Most of the saving of life was concentrated in the younger age groups, and took place during the 1740's and 1750's. Explanations in terms of increases in per capita consumption of food are obviously implausible for groups like the aristocracy and gentry, and given the age structure of the saving of life, we would expect a priori to find the reduction of childhood diseases to be implicated. Against this background, I have re-examined the literature on the history of inoculation against smallpox. No attempt is made to assess the magnitude of the latter's demographic consequences, as this must wait the fruits and results of work based on the new techniques and methods of historical demography.

To guide the reader through the somewhat confusing medical terminology and conflicting views on inoculation (variolation), and its relationship to vaccination, I now summarize the conventional medical position, followed by my own view. Inoculation is the injection of smallpox virus taken from a pustule of a person suffering from smallpox, whereas vaccination is the injection of virus taken originally from a cow suffering from cowpox. The two injections are distinguished by the symptoms and results that they produce: inoculation usually produces pustular eruptions around the body, typical of a mild form of smallpox, and is consequently infectious in that it spreads the disease to an unprotected population; vaccination produces only a local vesicle at the site of injection, which is not infectious. Both injections protect from future attacks of smallpox by eliciting the manufacture of antibodies within the person injected, which provide a defensive pool against future exposure to smallpox virus. Inoculation was first used by the medical profession in England in 1721, but was replaced by vaccination which was introduced by Edward Jenner in 1796. Vaccination, unlike inoculation, is a safe injection, both for the person injected and the unprotected population exposed to him, and this was the reason why inoculation was replaced by vaccination.

I have recently challenged this conventional medical view in a book on Edward Jenner's cowpox vaccine,[6] arguing that the vaccines used in Jenner's lifetime were in fact derived from smallpox virus, and that early vaccination was a form of inoculation. This conclusion undermines the polarisation of vaccination and inoculation, with the one being viewed as safe and effective, the other as dangerous and demographically damaging; it also raises the question as to the actual historical contribution of inoculation in reducing smallpox mortality. No-one has queried the prophylactic power of inoculation to protect against attacks of smallpox and it is generally agreed that being severer in its effects than vaccination, it produced a larger amount of antibody and a much longer period of immunity (usually for lifetime). The major argument against inoculation has always been that it spread smallpox to unprotected members of the population, because of its similarity to natural smallpox. We will see however that smallpox virus appears to have been attenuated by the process of inoculation, leading to negligible secondary contagion. Also, from a demographic point of view, it will be argued that secondary contagion was irrelevant on two grounds: (i) the universality of smallpox before the introduction of inoculation, virtually everyone in the population being affected by it; (ii) the danger of secondary infection led to the practice of general inoculation—all vulnerable members of a community being inoculated at one time—which resulted in a dramatic decline in smallpox mortality.

One final point on terminology: because of the development of inoculations for other diseases, the inoculation of smallpox virus is now known by the more specialised term of variolation. In this book, however, the term inoculation will continue to be employed as this was the term used by contemporaries in the eighteenth century, whose writings we will be referring to.

CHAPTER 1

Methods of Inoculation and Variations in the Severity of its Effects

The inoculation of smallpox is probably nearly as old as the disease itself, and reports of its existence appear in the literature as early as the late seventeenth century. It seems to have been a long-standing practice in China, India and parts of Arabia; in all these countries, inoculation was probably perfected over a period of hundreds of years. An English doctor living in India, J. Z. Holwell, described in 1767 a technique of inoculation which is remarkably similar to modern methods of vaccination:

"with a small instrument he [the Indian inoculator] wounds, by many slight touches, about the compass of a silver groat, just making the smallest appearance of blood, then . . . applies it [variolous matter] to the wound . . ."[7]

According to Holwell, the result was that "of the multitudes I have seen inoculated in that country, the number of pustules have seldom been less than fifty, and hardly ever exceeded two hundred", so that not "one in a million . . . miscarries under it."[8]

The inoculation of smallpox was also a part of the traditional folk medicine of Britain, but this only came to notice after Lady Mary Wortley Montagu had her daughter inoculated in London in 1721. Reports of folk inoculation appeared from Scotland and Wales, the latter giving rise to two independent accounts; Dr Perrot Williams described the history of the practice in Pembrokeshire:

"it has been commonly practised by the Inhabitants of this Part of Wales time out of mind, though by another Name, *viz* that of buying the Disease . . . In order to procure the Distemper to themselves, they either rub the Matter taken from the Pustules when ripe, on several Parts of the Skin of the Arms, etc or prick those Parts with Pins, or the like, first infected with the same Matter."[9]

This was confirmed by a Mr Richard Wright, a surgeon living in Haverford West, who interviewed a number of very old people in the area who said it had "been a common Practice with them time out of mind"[10]; one woman, a seventy-year midwife, stated that to her personal knowledge it had been practised "above fifty Years", and that she knew "but one dying" after the operation, in spite of "hundreds" having undergone it.[11]

"Buying the smallpox" was perhaps a more vivid way of describing the operation than the gardening metaphor "inoculation"—although the latter's meaning (transplantation), indicates the same contemporary belief that a favourable form of the disease was merely being transferred from one person to another. We will see later that this was a mistaken belief, and that the process of inoculation probably involved an attenuation of the virus.

The first medical account of inoculation to appear in England was that written by Dr Emanueli Timoni, an abstract of which was published in the *Philosophical Transactions* in 1714. Timoni, who practised medicine at Constantinople, claimed that of the "thousands" of people who had been inoculated during the previous eight years, "none have been found to die" of the operation.[12] He admitted however that occasionally symptoms were very severe, and in one year when smallpox was very fatal, four out of fifty cases had inoculated smallpox "near the confluent sort".[13] However, the suddeness of onset of the symptoms led to a suspicion that "these four had caught the common Small-Pox before the Incision was made"[14]—a problem which affected all forms of smallpox prophylaxsis, both inoculation and vaccination, in subsequent experience. Other than this complication, Timoni stated that the pustules resulting from inoculation were "distinct, few and scatter'd; commonly 10 or 20 break out; here and there one has but two or three, few have 100."[15] These very mild results from inoculation were almost certainly achieved through the technique of injection employed; Timoni described this as follows:

"the Operator is to make several little Wounds with a Needle, in one, two or more Places of the Skin, 'till some Drops of Blood follow, and immediately drop out some Drops of the Matter in the Glass, and mix it well with the Blood issuing out; one Drop of the Matter is sufficient for each Place pricked. These Punctures are made indifferently in any of the fleshy Parts, but succeed best in the Muscles of the Arm or Radius. The Needle is to be a three 'edged Surgeon's Needle; it may likewise be perform'd with a Lancet: The Custom is to run the Needle transverse, and rip up the skin a little, that there may be a convenient dividing of the Part, and the mixing of the Matter with the Blood more easily perform'd."[16]

The conclusions reached by Timoni about the safety and method of inoculation in Turkey, were confirmed by a number of independent witnesses, both medical and non-medical. Peter Kennedy, a Scottish surgeon who had practised at Constantinople, stated in a book written in 1715, that he had been informed by physicians and merchants living there, "that of the Number of two thousand, which had then lately undergone that Method [of inoculation], there were not any more than two who died."[17] Similarly, Dr Jacob Pylarini described in an account published in the *Philosophical Transactions* for 1716, how inoculation had been introduced into Turkey in 1701 from Thessaly, and described the method of inoculation as follows:

> "the Greek woman . . . pricks the middle of the Forehead, and the Temples at the Root of the Hairs; as also the Chin and both the Cheeks, with a steel or golden Needle, not thrusting it in straight, but obliquely, and separating the Skin a little with a sharp Point from the Flesh below. Then with the same Needle she introduces the Pus into the little Orifices, and ties a Bandage over the Parts . . . The Eruption is almost always of the **distinct** kind, and the Pustules not numerous; but frequently twenty or thirty, rarely a hundred, and very seldom two hundred."[13]

The injection in the forehead, chin, cheeks etc, was a residue of the Christian belief that incisions made in the pattern of a cross would help to ensure their success, but although we would find this aspect of the practice quaint, the actual technique of inoculation appears to have been very sound, with very good results.

It was soon after Pylarini gave his account of inoculation, that Lady Mary Wortley Montagu wrote her famous letter to a friend in 1717, describing her observations of inoculation in Constantinople when she was the wife of the English ambassador:

> "The smallpox, so fatal, and so general amongst us, is here [Constantinople] entirely harmless, by the invention of in grafting [inoculation], which is the term they give it. There is a set of old women, who make it their business to perform the operation, every autumn in the month of September, when the great heat is abated . . . the old woman comes with a nutshell full of the matter of the best sort of smallpox, and asks what vein you please to have opened. She immediately opens that you offer her, with a large needle (which gives you no more pain than a common scratch) and puts into the vein, as much matter as can lie upon the head of her needle, and after that binds up the little wound with a hollow bit of shell; and in this manner opens four or five veins . . . The children or young patients play together all the rest of the day, and are in perfect health to the eighth. Then the fever begins to seize them, and they keep their beds two days, very seldom three. They have very rarely above twenty or thirty [pustules] in their faces, which never mark, and in eight days they are as well as before their illness . . . Every year thousands undergo this operation, and the French Ambassador says pleasantly that they take the smallpox here by way of diversion, as they take waters

in other countries. There is no example of anyone that has died in it . . ."[19]

Lady Montagu was almost certainly wrong in stating that virus was inoculated into veins—no other account mentions such a practice, and there are virological grounds for believing it to be unlikely—and she appears to have glossed over some of the complications known to have arisen on occasions with inoculation, such as those mentioned by Timoni. Nevertheless, her overall account is compatible with the numerous other ones of Turkish inoculation, and there is no doubt that she herself was an eye-witness to most of what she described.

The mildness of inoculation in Turkey was further confirmed by Charles Maitland, who was surgeon to the British Embassy at the time Lord Montagu was ambassador: "The Pustules, whether many or few (and they commonly were from 10 to 100, sometimes more) never left any Marks or Pits behind them, except only in the Incisions, or Parts Ingrafted."[20] Maitland was present and assisted in the inoculation of Lady Mary Montagu's son at Constantinople in 1717; his account of this second known inoculation of English children (two children of an Embassy official had been previously inoculated) is not only of historical interest, but marks the beginning of a practice that had a serious and long-lasting effect on the history of inoculation in England itself:

"She [Lady Montagu] . . . sent for an old Greek Woman, who had practised this Way a great many Years . . . but so awkwardly by the shaking of her Hand, and put the Child to so much Torture with her blunt and rusty Needle, that I pitied his Cries, who had ever been of such Spirit and Courage, that hardly any Thing of Pain could make him cry before; and therefore Inoculated the other Arm with my own Instrument [lancet], and with so little Pain to him, that he did not in the least complain of it."[20]

From the very beginning of the practice of inoculation by the English medical profession, a lancet rather than a needle was used, and this affected the depth with which incisions were made, at least until Robert Sutton restored the practice of slight incisions in the late 1750s. It was only in this century, that the advantages of a needle over a lancet were realised for the purposes of vaccination by the medical profession, even though the more astute practitioners of folk medicine had realised this at a very early stage. When Dr P. Russel described the method of inoculation to a group of Turkish women at the end of the 1750s, his account was commended by an old Bedouin female servant who had herself inoculated a large number of people, except that he "did not seem so well to understand the way of performing the operation, which she asserted should be done not with a lancet, but with a needle."[21] One of the problems was that the medical profession found it difficult to accept that this radically effective prophylactic technique against smallpox had not been discovered by one of their own members, but by people with no pretension to the conventional medical wisdom of the day. The defensiveness of the medical profession sometimes resulted in extreme arrogance, so that one of the earliest opponents of inoculation could say that the practice of a "few ignorant women . . . so far obtains in one of the politest nations in the world, as to be received in the Royal Palace."[22] In fact most of the innovations in the technique of inoculation came from obscure surgeons and what contemporaries contemptuously sometimes referred to as "empirics"; this is probably just one example in the history of medicine of how really important practical medical discoveries have occurred through empirical observation or chance, rather than theoretical understanding. To this day, we do not fully understand the immunology of either inoculation or vaccination, in spite of their enormous historical practical importance.

The success of the practice of inoculation in Turkey was further confirmed in 1722 by Dr James Jurin, secretary to the Royal Society, but he brought out the importance of a particular inoculator for the history of inoculation in that country:

"out of many thousands that in the space of about forty years past have been inoculated in and about Constantinople by one Greek woman, who still continues that Practice notwithstanding her extreme old age, not so much as one Person has miscarried, as I am assured by the igenious Dr Le Duc, a Native of Constantinople who was himself inoculated there under the Care of his Father, an eminent Physician in that City."[23]

According to Porter in 1755, this woman came from Morea, and was succeeded by a woman from Bosnia; apparently inoculation was only practiced on a very limited scale in Turkey and thus the importance of these individual inoculators.[24]

There were other inoculators in Constantinople, but it appears that at least one of them was very much less successful than the women from Morea and Bosnia. Details of this unsuccessful technique are of some importance for understanding the history of inoculation, and were revealed in an extract from a letter written by Timoni published in 1734:

"at the beginning of the practice of inoculation of the smallpox at Constantinople, there was a person who used to make an incision through the skin, and then introduce into the wound the scab of a dried pustule, tying a bandage over it . . . this mode of operating was objectionable, not only on account of the pain attending it, but also because it sometimes excited the small-pox in its worst form, while at other times it failed to communicate the disease, though even then it produced very bad sores in the places where the incisions had been made. Moreover in some instances this mode of inoculation terminated fatally."[25]

The reasons for the relative failure of this type of inoculation will be discussed later; here it is sufficient to note that the depth of the injection was probably a factor.

The first inoculation of a known individual in England was of Lady Montagu's daughter in April 1721, which was performed by Maitland in London. This was successful and the patient had less than one hundred pustules as a result of her inoculation.[26] Maitland was very important in the introduction of inoculation into England and he was responsible for the experimental inoculation of the six Newgate prisoners in the autumn of 1721, the success of which helped to persuade the royal family and the aristocracy to have their own children inoculated. Unfortunately, Maitland left no account of his technique but it is almost certain that he made deep incisions with a lancet; he described how typically the incisions he made led to "a vast Discharge" of matter,[27] a symptom known to be associated with deep injections. This conclusion is confirmed by an eye-witness account of Maitland's inoculations of the Newgate prisoners: "The Incisions were long and large."[28] The result of this method was much severer than that practised by the Greek women in Turkey; several children had 300 pustules and more, while one had "above two Thousand".[29] This was the beginning of a fairly severe form of inoculation, which was used by all practitioners in Britain until the innovation of Robert Sutton in the late 1750s. It seriously checked the practice of inoculation, as people feared that either they or their children would die from the operation.

There were two main reasons why the early British inoculators adopted the deep injection technique: an anxiety about whether inoculation would actually produce a form of smallpox (some contemporaries questioned whether the light Turkish form would achieve this[30]), and the belief that the "poison" of smallpox had to be discharged through an "issue" for a successful outcome. The latter was a part of a long-held humoral theory of smallpox, which assumed that everyone inherited the "seeds" of the disease, which had to be expressed through the eruption of smallpox before true health could be achieved. Some of the early inoculators claimed however, that the deeper injections were also more successful because of the copious discharge at the site of the incision, than were the lighter forms of inoculation; for example, Nettleton who was one of the first to practice inoculation on any scale wrote in 1722:

> "I generally found, that in those who discharged most this way, the Fever was more slight, and the **Small Pox** fewer, tho' I have known some do very well when these places have only appeared very red, but have scarce run any thing at all, as it usually happens, when the Incision is made so superficial as not to cut thro' the Skin."[31]

This conclusion was based however on only forty cases, and the lack of any systematic experimental evidence meant that Nettleton could in effect assert opposite propositions in the same sentence, without feeling a need to further clarify the position. Contemporaries were predisposed to accept the conclusion about the benefits of deep incisions because of their theoretical beliefs; Rogers summarized the consensus of opinion on this subject in his book on epidemic diseases published in 1734:

> " 'Tis observed, the more these Incisions discharge, during the Course of the Disease, the more gentle all the Symptoms are; and the longer they continue open, the more perfect Health the Patient enjoys afterwards . . . Part of the morbid **Virus**, must be supposed to be thrown out from the circulating Juices . . ."[32]

Again this conclusion was based on a very limited number of cases—there were only 897 inoculations performed in the whole of Great Britain, the American colonies and Hanover in the period 1721-28[33]—and later experience was to show how false it was.

The actual depth of the incisions made in this early period was indicated by a number of authors during the 1720s. Henry Newman described how in New England, "we make usually a Couple of Incisions in the Arms where we make our Issues, but somewhat larger than for them, sometimes in one Arm, and one leg."[34] Boylston confirmed this, and gave advice on how inoculation should be performed:

> "Let the Incisions be made with a good Lancet thro' the true Skin [dermis], (by pinching of it up between your Fingers) across the Fibres, and about a quarter of an Inch long, such as would receive a common Pea in case you were to make an Issue . . ."[35]

An even more detailed description of technique was given by Claudius Amyand, the King's surgeon, in a letter written at the beginning of 1724:

> "all my operations have been performed with a Lancet on the brawny parts of the two Arms into the Cutis [dermis]

and sometimes beyond it. The Incisions have been sometimes an Inch long and sometimes only the length of a Barley-Corn and so superficial as not to penetrate the Cutis, and the Consequences have been much the same."[86]

Unfortunately, Amyand did not realise that the crucial point concerned not only the depth of the injection into the dermis and beyond, but also whether the injection penetrated fully into the dermis itself; it was only later with the innovation in technique made by Robert Sutton, that the importance of not going beyond the boundary between the epidermis and dermis was realised.

Lady Mary Wortley Montagu was aware of the dangers of the departure from the Turkish method of inoculation and complained that "the miserable gashes that they [the English inoculators] give people in the arms may endanger the loss of them."[87] The English medical profession itself realised some of the problems that very deep injections created, for in 1736 Sir Hans Sloane warned that "great care should be had in making the incision, not to go thro' the skin; for in that case I have seen it attended with very troublesome consequences afterwards."[88] Burges later claimed that the dangers of really deep injections—penetrating through the dermis so as to wound the "cellular membrane"—were discovered by Ranby; he described the symptomatic advantages of the new technique as follows:

"In the infancy of the practice, it was the custom to cut the incision through the skin into the cellular membrane, from a prejudice then generally established, that one of the advantages of inoculation was securing a drain for the humours by the wound, which in that case generally continued its discharge for a considerable time after the distemper was over. But it was found that the incision which was at first only considered as an issue, was too often attended with several very troublesome symptoms, such as an inflammation and swelling of the whole arm, which was reduced with many difficulties, the wound continuing a troublesome sore to the surgeon, and a painful one to the patient a long time . . . Besides, it was no unusual thing at the same time for the person to be seized with other inflammatory disorders, that seemed to point out the cause and seat of the evil."[89]

The advantage claimed for the new lighter method of inoculation was that it led to less soreness at the site of injection, and fewer inflammatory complications; nowhere in the literature is it stated that the severity of the inoculated smallpox— the number of pustules etc—was affected. Burges gives the somewhat misleading impression that the newer lighter method was universally adopted by all inoculators; this was not the case. A Dr Henry Barnes who practised at Carlisle, gave the following account of his method of inoculation in 1755:

"I always chuse to make the Incision so deep as to pierce the Skin quite thro' to the Membrana Adiposa, allowing the Incision to bleed for a few minutes, then the running of the Blood may not wash away the infected matter."[40]

Barnes claimed that his method was highly successful, and that of the "near four hundred" that had been inoculated in the Carlisle area by him, not one had died.[41] This claim was probably correct, but undoubtedly the symptoms resulting from his inoculations were at least as severe as those of Sloane, Ranby and others who adopted the somewhat lighter method. The key change in technique and resulting symptomology occurred with the Suttons, as we shall now see.

Robert Sutton was a surgeon practising in Suffolk and he appears to have started practice as an inoculator in about 1757.. He first announced his new method of inoculation in the *Ipswich Journal* on the 1st May 1762, claiming that "his new Method of inoculating for the Small-Pox, which he has used for these four Months past, has succeeded so well, that upwards of Two hundred Patients have not had, upon an Average, a hundred Pustules each."[42] Later in the same year, on the 25th September, he gave the following account of his new method:

"Robert Sutton, Surgeon, of Kenton in Suffolk, continues to carry on his new Method of Inoculation with the greatest Success; and being done without Incision, the most curious Eye cannot discern where the Operation is performed for the first forty-eight Hours . . . He has inoculated since December last, three hundred and sixty five . . ."[43]

Although Sutton used a lancet rather than a needle, his technique appears to have been almost identical to that practised in Turkey. Very little further information on Robert Sutton's practice is available in the literature, as it was his son Daniel Sutton, who publicized and was responsible for making the new method widely known. There has been some confusion about the relative roles of father and son in making the innovation of technique, but its clear from contemporary accounts of Daniel Sutton's practice that he was merely following his father's methods. Robert Houlton confirmed this in two separate publications—Daniel Sutton used a "puncture so slight, that it is scarce felt by the patient, and which in a minute afterwards is scarce visible."[44] "The operation is performed on most without their feeling or knowing it: and in a minute afterwards, the puncture is scarce visible."[45]

Daniel Sutton himself described his method as follows: "The lancet being charged with the smallest perceivable quantity (and the smaller the better) of unripe, crude or watery matter, immediately introduce it by puncture, obliquely, between the scarf [epidermis] and true skin [dermis], barely sufficient to draw blood."[46]

Although the Sutton family had attempted to keep their method a secret, contemporaries had soon discovered its essence through questioning patients and others who had witnessed the practice (this was made all the easier through the large number of partnerships with outsiders that the Suttons formed). Thomas Dimsdale was perhaps one of the most important inoculators to publish details on the new method; his book, *The Present Method of Inoculating for the Smallpox*, written at the end of 1766, went into several editions and described two variations on the new technique:

"an incision is made in that part of the arm where issues are usually placed, deep enough to pass through the scarf skin [epidermis], and just to touch the skin itself [dermis], and in length as short as possible, not more than one eighth of an inch . . . I have also tried the following method, with the same success as that above described . . . A lancet being moistened with the variolous fluid in the same manner as in the other, is gently introduced in an oblique manner between the scarf and true skin . . ."[47]

The essence of the difference between this new method and that practised by British inoculators since the 1730s, was brought out by William Bromfield, an opponent of the Suttonian innovation:

"I will not insist on it that matter introduced between the cuticle [epidermis] and cutis [dermis] is not equally capable of producing the disease as where a scratch is made thro' the same integument sufficient to slightly wound the true skin [dermis] . . . [which is the method] that of late years has been practised . . ."[48]

Given that it became universally accepted that the Suttonian method was the key innovation in technique, it is clear that much lighter effects were produced by injecting virus into the epidermis or, at most, the boundary between the epidermis and dermis, rather than fully into the dermis itself. I will discuss possible virological explanations of this conclusion in a later chapter.

Although contemporaries generally acknowledged the success of the Suttonian method, few realised the critical importance of the depth of the injection. There were even some inoculators who continued to operate in the old way; for example, the Rev. James Woodforde noted in his diary for the 22nd November, 1776, how an amateur inoculator by the name of Drake made "a deep incision in both arms."[49] This was almost certainly untypical at this time, and Woodforde describes what was a more orthodox method in giving an account of the inoculation of two of his servants by Dr Thorne of Mattishall in the same year:

"the Dr. taking a small bit of Cotton Thread saturated with Matter between his Left hand Finger and Thumb with the Launcett in his other hand, he then dipt the Point of the Launcett in a Tea Cup of warm water, then rubbed the Launcett in the Cotton Thread and with the Point of the Launcett made two dotts like this: about two Inches apart in each of their arms . . . scarce to be felt or draw blood, they then stood with their arms exposed to the cold air for about three minutes, till almost dried up: the Matter took effect almost instantaneously, and plain to be seen, the Place where the Dots were made was a little above the other Flesh, like a small sting of a Nettle—No Plaister or anything else whatever put to their arms afterwards . . ."[50]

Up until the Suttonian innovation, it had been standard practice to apply a plaister because of the depth of injections, but this was abandoned with the lighter technique.

The person who came nearest to realising the key importance of the depth of injection in the Suttonian method was, ironically, Edward Jenner. In his first publication on his new cowpox inoculation in 1798, he gave the following conclusion, based on many years experience of smallpox inoculation:

"I have the strongest reason for supposing that if either the punctures or incisions be made so deep as to go through it [the skin], and wound the adipose membrane, that the risk of bringing on a violent disease is greatly increased. I have known an inoculator, whose practice was 'to cut deep enough (to use his own expression) to see a bit of fat', and there to lodge the matter. The great number of bad Cases, independent of inflammations and abscesses on the arms, and the fatality which attended this practice was almost inconceivable . . . It was the practice of another, whom I well remember, to pinch up a small portion of the skin on the arms of his patients and to pass through it a needle, with a thread attached to it previously dipped in variolous matter. The thread was lodged in the perforated part, and consequently left in contact with the cellular membrane. This practice was attended with the same ill success as the former . . . A very respectable friend of mine, Dr Hardwicke, of Sodbury in this county [Gloucestershire] inoculated great numbers of patients previous to the introduction of the more moderate method by Sutton, and with such success, that a fatal instance occurred as rarely as since that method has been adopted. It was the doctor's practice to make as slight an incision as possible **upon** the skin, and there to lodge a thread saturated with the variolous matter."[51]

Although Jenner did not distinguish carefully enough between the effects of wounding the "adipose membrane" ("inflammations and abcesses on the arms") and the results of injecting virus into the dermis and beyond ("fatality which attended this practice"), he came nearest to any of his contemporaries in realising the relationship between depth of injection and the success of inoculation. By the end of the eighteenth century however, most inoculators did practice the Suttonian method of inoculation; this was acknowledged by Jenner when he referred to the demise of the old method: "it is very improbable that any one would now inoculate in this rude way by design."[52]

The impact of technique on the safety of inoculation is obviously critical in assessing its historical significance. However, there is one major obstacle which must be surmounted before we can discuss the evidence on the severity of inoculated smallpox: the problem of inoculated people catching natural smallpox before their inoculation. We have already noted how Timoni had experienced this difficulty when attempting to assess the effects of inoculation in Turkey, and it was a problem for anyone attempting to evaluate any form of smallpox prophylaxsis—inoculation or vaccination. British and European inoculators considerably compounded this problem by introducing a lengthy period of medical preparation before inoculation—a period which obviously left those to be inoculated vulnerable to natural infection, particularly during the time of a smallpox epidemic. Angelo Gatti—who had witnessed the practice of inoculation in Turkey and had closely observed its subsequent history in Europe—wrote in 1766 an account of how the European inoculators introduced the practice of preparation:

> "Ever since inoculation has been received in Europe, the practitioners have been of the opinion that the essential advantages of artificial and natural smallpox were, 1. the preparation; 2. the discharge of the variolous matter by means of the wounds; 3. the assistance of art in a disorder which is known as soon as it appears. All inoculators have said, prepare your subjects; procure an outlet to the venom; be attentive to administer every help of art, when the disorder shews itself."[53]

The major reason for the introduction of medical preparation again appears to have been due to a belief in humoral pathology, although Lady Montagu strongly implied that it was very much in the medical profession's economic interest to bring about this innovation.[54] There was no single systematic and consistent body of beliefs on the humoral pathology of smallpox which can be quoted from the literature, but James Burges came nearest to justifying preparation in these terms, in his treatise published in 1764:

> "and what makes it [smallpox] still more dreadful is, that the poison lies concealed in the blood, while perhaps the unhappy subject, ignorant of the approaching calamity, is urging the latent venom into action, and rendering his constitution unequal to the attack . . . when the skin is . . . obstructed, that the matter cannot find a passage through its pores, and nature wants force to bring on a proper suppuration, the infectious particles being reabsorbed by the blood, occasion those obstructions in the smaller vessels, that generally end in mortification . . . preparation [ensures] . . . that it [the patient's body] is neither too low to support the attack of the infection, or so loaded and overcharged as to obstruct the expulsion of it, or so heated as to conspire with the malady in raising the flame to too great a heighth."[55]

There are inconsistent elements in this passage, but what emerges centrally is a notion of "constitutions" which are too "high"—inflaming the virulence of the disease by energising it—or too "low", so as to be incapable of expelling the illness. In practice, Burges like his contemporaries appears to have been most concerned with constitutions which were too high and he noted that "in very lax habits, such as children, and delicate young women, the hazard is less, as such constitutions are in some degree in a natural state of preparation."[56] Constitutions which were thought to be too high were robust and active ones, and the disease was believed to be inflamed by animal foods—but reduced by purging, bleeding and a vegetarian diet.

Preparation therefore took the form of purging, bleeding and restriction to a low diet, and these are measures which were used by the medical profession in the treatment of natural smallpox before the advent of inoculation. Maitland very quickly resorted to dietary measures in the treatment of his inoculated cases,[57] and Nettleton, who published next to him, "employed a preparatory treatment of emetics, purgatives, and sometimes bleeding" and required patients to "abstain from animal foods and strong liquors."[58] This period of preparation soon became a lengthy affair, and Rogers writing in 1734, referred to the "necessary Preparations for about three Weeks Diet and Medicine."[59] There was a tendency for this period of preparation to lengthen, and when Edward Jenner was inoculated as a boy in 1756, he underwent, according to one of his early biographers, the following experience:

"This preparation lasted six weeks. He was bled, to ascertain whether his blood was fine; was purged repeatedly, till he became emaciated and feeble; was kept on a very low diet, small in quantity, and dosed with a diet-drink to sweeten the blood."[60]

We must allow for some exaggeration in this account, as it was written by someone concerned to discredit inoculation, but it probably contains the substance of truth about the length and nature of preparation. The medical profession soon appears however to have realised the irrelevance of much of the preparatory measures, and Monro writing in 1765 about the history of inoculation in Scotland stated:

"When inoculation was first introduced into this country, those who were to undergo it were prepared for the operation by blood letting, purgatives, aperients and low diet: but the gentlemen of practice observing that the eruption did not proceed so well in children thus weakened, as in those who had undergone evacuations, they are now generally omitted; and a mild cooling diet to the patient, or its nurse, with a genteel laxative to empty the intestines, are the principal preparations."[61]

This simplification of preparation does not seem however to have led to a shortening of the time involved, for it would appear that before Daniel Sutton reduced the period of preparation in his practice, this still took "from a month, which then was the usual time."[62]

Such a long period of preparation obviously exposed patients to great potential dangers, particularly during smallpox epidemics. This was unintentionally revealed in an account of a very malignant smallpox epidemic in Blandford, Dorset in 1766, when "a perfect rage for inoculation seized the town."[63] This mass inoculation was widely publicised because of the relatively high proportion of people dying from smallpox after inoculation; a local doctor in describing the "ill success of inoculation" noted that

"out of 384, who lately inoculated at Blandford, 150 were poor people, for whom the parish paid the operations. Not one of these had the confluent smallpox; not one died. Of the rest a great number were in danger from confluent smallpox; and thirteen died . . . a preparatory course was despised . . . the impatience of some was so great, that they left their accustomed apothecaries for the sake of being inoculated a day or two sooner."[64]

The writer of this account tried to blame the high proportion of severe cases on the negligence of preparation, but the very opposite appears to have been the case. The impatient people were those with **accustomed apothecaries,** and it would have been this group that would have received conventional preparation. No mention is made of the preparation of the 150 poor people, and this is probably because the parish was unwilling to pay the relatively high cost of full preparation. Ironically, it was the richer parishioners, who could afford the cost of full preparation, who were most vulnerable to catching natural smallpox before the effects of inoculation had time to take place. The point must not be exaggerated as smallpox spreads relatively slowly from person to person—it was often present in market towns for up to two years before it had exhausted the available supply of victims.

The first inoculator to completely dispense with preparation was a surgeon by the name of Williams. At the end of 1768 he placed the following advertisement in the *Northampton Mercury:*

"INOCULATION WITHOUT PREPARATION (Established by a five years successful Experience, commonly called the Williams Short Method). Mr Williams . . . and a Number of Partners, have inoculated and lightly carried through many thousand persons without the usual tedious and too often injurious preparative Treatment by very strict Diet and strong Mercurial Purges . . ."[65]

Two years after this advertisement Williams died, for at Kibworth, a large village about ten miles from Leicester, on the western wall of the Church is the following inscription:

"In Memory of Mr Lewis Paul Williams, Surgeon. He departed this life January 9th 1771, in his 40th year. He was the first that introduced into practice Inoculation without preparation into this Kingdom."[66]

According to Williams' own advertisement, he first dispensed with preparation in 1763, at about the same time as Daniel Sutton began to shorten the period of preparation in his practice. Williams had much less direct influence than the Suttons, for his name never appeared in any contemporary medical works on inoculation or smallpox. However, as his monument implied, others soon followed him and these others may have been influenced by Williams or his partners. His innovation, like that of the Suttons, was merely a return to the Turkish practice and in one sense an inevitable logical development towards the complete simplification of inoculation.

According to Woodville, Daniel Sutton broke away from his father partly on grounds of disagreement about the period of necessary preparation, Daniel proposing to "reduce the process preparatory to inoculation, from a month, which then was the usual time, to eight or ten days."[67] Because of the eventual popularity of the Suttonian method, this innovation had great importance in reducing preparation, although it is clear that a number of other inoculators quite independently came to the conclusion that preparation was entirely irrelevant to the success of inoculation. Andrew noted in 1765 that

"the little Necessity there is for Preparation is confirmed by the Account I received lately from Dr Swan, of Newcastle, who informs me that in his Neighbourhood 70 or 80 Persons were Inoculated without the least Preparation, and all recovered of the Small-Pox."[68]

This type of empirical observation led to the inevitable conclusion, and Dimsdale in his highly popular book on inoculation of 1767 also came near to reaching it:

"That [improvement] which appears most likely to be made, is in shortening the time of preparation; for as I have often been obliged to inoculate without any, and have always had the same success, it has inclined me to think, that much, if not the whole of this process may be dispensed with (except in very full habits, or where other particular circumstances require it)."[69]

And in the same year, Watts came to a similar conclusion, based on the experience of a friend who was a surgeon who "began to inoculate without any previous preparation at all."[70]

To a very large extent, inoculators were forced to abandon preparation because of the reactions of their patients. We have already seen how people in Blandford had become impatient at the delay in becoming inoculated, and a similar thing occurred at Witham, Essex in 1779 when "the great mortality which attended the natural smallpox, induced many of the inhabitants to be inoculated . . . in less than a week, upwards of one thousand persons were inoculated without any previous preparation whatever."[71] Similarly, many of the 928 poor people inoculated at Luton in 1788, refused to take their preparatory medicines, in spite of having promised to do so.[72] By 1796, Daniel Sutton could note that "it has been a practice of late, to give up preparation, medicinal and dietetic entirely."[73] However, some more conventional practitioners were reluctant to entirely abandon preparation, and as late as 1797 Woodville lamented "the ignorant and foolish parents who were unwilling to subject their children to the necessary preparation."[74] He linked this to the decline of the use of special isolation houses in which patients underwent preparation; in fact, these houses could be a considerable source of danger to patients during an epidemic, as was shown by the following experience in Hastings:

"In this year [1796-97] the disease [smallpox] was prevalent in all districts round Hastings, and inoculation was general amongst all classes; houses being specially set up for reception of the patients . . . In these three months [Dec. 1796-March 1797] 11 persons are stated to have 'died of smallpox in the natural way' and 61 'in consequence of inoculation'."[75]

This high mortality amongst inoculated people was virtually unknown in a normal situation, and it is almost certain that most of the inoculated people dying from smallpox in Hastings caught the disease during the period of preparation while living in the isolation houses. All this is yet a further example of how the medical profession had difficulty in seeing what was obvious to many other people because of their attachment to the notions of contemporary conventional medical wisdom; Woodville's arrogant dismissal of "the ignorant and foolish parents" who ignored preparatory measures, was echoed by a conventional surgeon who complained in 1800 that

"whenever the inoculating rage once takes place, whole parishes are doomed, without the least attention to age, sex, or temperament—no previous preparation, no after-treatment or concern . . . Are not scores and hundreds seized upon at once, for the insidious scratchings, puncturings and threadings, without ever a possibility of their being attended to?"[76]

Much inoculation at this time was beginning to be undertaken by amateur inoculators and even parents themselves, and the outrage felt by a member of the medical profession whose conventional medical skills were being made redundant, can be felt across the nearly two intervening centuries.

Given the variations in technique and methods of preparation discussed so far in this chapter, the evaluation of the severity of the symptoms resulting from inoculation, obviously becomes difficult. A review of the literature nevertheless does lead to certain firm conclusions, but these must always set in the context of the various complicating factors already discussed.

There are two major ways of evaluating the severity of inoculation: (i) the number of pustules, amount of fever and other symptoms of smallpox; (ii) the proportion of people dying after inoculation. I shall discuss these in sequence, but under the separate headings. From the very beginning, European inoculators noted the more severe symptoms of their inoculations compared to that of the Turkish experience. Newman, an English lawyer who had witnessed the practice of variolation in New England, wrote in 1722:

"The Number of the **Pustules** is not alike in all, in some they are a **very few**, in others they amount to an **Hundred**, in many they amount unto **several Hundreds**; frequently unto more than what the Accounts from the **Levant** say is usual there."[77]

This conclusion is confirmed by the more detailed literature on the number of pustules resulting from inoculation; Robert Waller, an apothecary who practised variolation in Gosport in Hampshire in 1722 and 1723, gave a list of the number of pustules in his inoculated cases as follows:

"1. Thirty. 2. Thirty. 3. About Twenty. 4. Some Thousands. 5. Four Or Five Hundred, Not To Be Numbered. 6. Fifty. 7. Six Or Seven Hundred. 8. Two Thousand. 9. Four Or Five Hundred. 10. About A Hundred. 11. Fifteen Hundred. 12. Fifteen Hundred. 13. Two Hundred. 14. Fifteen Or Twenty And But Small Ones. 15. Fifteen Or Twenty Little Ones. 16. The Confluent Kind All Over Her, With Many Purple Spots (And Died On The Tenth Day After She Was Inoculated). 17. Two Thousand."[78]

The variation in the number of pustules seems to have been partly a function of differences in technique used by Waller—the cases with the smallest number of pustules appearing to be those where the lightest incisions were made—but the important overall conclusion to emerge from this list, is the much greater severity of symptoms than reported from Turkey, and to be later found with the Suttonian method. Claudius Amyand, who was the royal surgeon at this time, gave a very detailed account of both his technique (as we have seen) and the resulting symptoms in his patients. His deep incisions resulted in the following numbers of pustules amongst his inoculated cases: 150, about 300, some thousands, 12, less than 20, 200, about 200, above 500, "many more than could be numbered".[79]

The greater severity of inoculation in Britain after its introduction in 1721, and before the innovation of technique made by Robert Sutton, is confirmed by a number of authors writing of the contrast between the pre- and post-Suttonian period. For example, Dr Giles Watts writing in 1767 stated:

"A few years ago, he had two of his sons inoculated by a very judicious and experienced practitioner, in the old way. One of them had the confluent small-pox, and hardly, very hardly, escaped with life; and the other too had the distemper very severely. He has often visited patients under inoculation in the old way. And he does not remember, that he ever knew a company of ten or a dozen inoculated together in that way, but one, or more of the company has had the distemper in a pretty severe manner. Very lately he has had four of his

family inoculated in the new way, and all of them together
have not had so many as eighty pustules."[80]

Similarly, Dimsdale writing in the same year, concluded:

"A considerable share of employment in this branch of my
profession has for upwards of twenty years occurred to me;
and altho' I have been fortunate as not to lose a patient
under inoculation, except one person, about fourteen years
ago, who after the eruption of a few distinct pustules died
of a fever, which I esteemed wholly independent of the
small-pox, yet I must acknowledge that in some cases the
symptoms have cost me not a little anxiety for the event . . .
such who were treated in . . . [the new] way, passed thro'
the distemper in a more favourable manner, than my own
patients, or those of the most able practitioners in the old
method of inoculation."[81]

We are fortunate to have a very exact account of the
number of pustules resulting from the Suttonian method of
inoculation from the report of a series of experiments published
by Dr William Watson in 1768. Watson was responsible for medical treatment of children in the Foundling Hospital, and decided
in 1767 to conduct a trial experiment using the Suttonian method
on the children in his care. Although we find this willingness to
experiment on children rather shocking—and this was common
practice amongst Watson's contemporaries—it has the advantage
for the medical historian of providing information under more
controlled conditions than is usual with most of the literature
considered. As these children were not inoculated as a result of a
threat of an epidemic, it removed the risk of prior infection with
natural smallpox, and provides a classic and exact account of the
effects of Suttonian inoculation. Altogether, 74 children were
inoculated, the lancet being "obliquely directed, that the matter
might be inserted between the cuticle and the skin"—and as was
standard Suttonian practice, no plaister was used to cover the
punctures made in each arm.[82] These 74 children had a total of
2,364, an average of 32 pustules each; three cases had a significantly greater number of pustules than average—440,260 and 200—
and excluding these three cases gives an average of just over 20
pustules per case.[83] It will be noted by comparing these figures
with those quoted in connection with Waller's and Amyand's early
practice, that the Suttonian method had dramatically reduced
the severity of symptoms, even amongst those with the greatest
number of pustules. In fact the Suttons were probably achieving
even milder results than the average in Watson's experiment, as
there were significant variations depending upon the type of
smallpox matter used for inoculation. Daniel Sutton advocated
the use of "unripe, crude or watery matter"[84] *i.e.* material taken

at an early stage of the development of a smallpox pustule—and Watson found that this was the only factor of all that he examined that made any difference to the outcome of severity. The 31 cases inoculated with watery matter had a total of 428 pustules—an average of just under fourteen each, the most of any single case being "near two hundred"—whereas as the remaining 43 cases inoculated with purulent or concocted matter, had a total of 1,936 pustules, an average of about forty-five each.[85]

As we have seen earlier, not all inoculators adopted the Suttonian innovation of technique after it had been introduced. This meant that some of them were still producing fairly severe results well after the late 1760s; for example, the Rev. Woodforde noted in his diary on the 8th May, that of the four Custance children inoculated by Dr William Downe at Norwich, two of them had the smallpox "pretty full".[86] This was probably fairly exceptional by this time, as the Suttons had forced their rivals to adopt their methods through the competitive process of the market.[87] Of course the Suttons were in the main only returning to the original simple method of inoculation practised in Turkey, India and elsewhere—in effect undoing the damage done by the medical profession—but they must be credited for having paid very close attention to their experience, and working within the best English empirical tradition.

The reduction in severity of symptoms from inoculation was mirrored in the decline of mortality rates from the operation. The inquiry sponsored by the Royal Society into the relative safety of inoculation had yielded a figure of seventeen people dying out of the 827 people inoculated in 1721-28, *i.e.* nearly two per cent.[88] Dr James Jurin, who was mainly responsible for compiling the statistics, noted the complication referred to earlier, of people catching smallpox before they were inoculated, and quoted in particular the experience of the New England inoculators, who had inoculated as a result of an epidemic:

> "The Reverend Mr Mather, in a Letter dated March 10 1721 from Boston in New England, gives an Account, That of near 300 inoculated there, 5 or 6 died upon it or after it, but from other Diseases and Accidents, chiefly from having taken the Infection in the common way, before it could be given them in this way of Transplantation."[89]

Jurin included five of these deaths in the list of those who died from inoculation in order "to avoid all occasion of dispute"[90], and so it is clear that these early figures on the effects of inoculation overstated its dangers. Some of the deaths however would almost certainly have been due to the inoculation itself, and this comes out through a consideration of specially vulnerable categories of people. Infants and pregnant women were generally recognized as being especially vulnerable to inoculation; when

2,000 people were inoculated in the Hampshire/Sussex/Surrey area in 1740, two of them died—both pregnant women[91] and of 1,215 people inoculated at Luton in 1788, five died all under the age of four months.[92] These two examples illustrate that inoculation could kill directly, particularly these vulnerable types of people.

The mortality rate amongst the 2,000 people inoculated in the Hampshire/Sussex/Surrey region—one per cent—seems to have been fairly typical of the pre-Suttonian era. Of 5,554 people inoculated in Scotland up until 1765, 72 died, giving a mortality rate of 1.3 per cent.[93] The inoculation mortality rate in Boston, New England can be traced in some detail because of the precise historical information which is available: 2.0 per cent in 1721, 3.0 per cent in 1730, 1.4 per cent in 1752, and 0.9 per cent in 1764.[94] Although some of these rates are based on several thousands of cases, they cannot be taken literally, as most inoculations in Boston were undertaken because of the existence of epidemics; also, inoculation was banned by law in Boston in the absence of an epidemic, and there would have been an inevitably large number of cases of people catching natural smallpox before resorting to panic inoculations. Individual English practitioners claimed much greater success in their private practice, and this may have been a genuine function of not having to inoculate people so frequently as a panic measure during epidemics. Andrew claimed in 1765 that he had inoculated more than three hundred people in the Exeter area during the previous twenty-three years, "not one of whom has miscarried; and in my whole Practice I have only lost one."[95] As we have seen, Dimsdale gave an account of an almost identical degree of success during the twenty years and more practice of inoculation ("I have been so fortunate as not to lose a patient under inoculation, except one person, about fourteen years ago, who after the eruption of a few distinct pustules died of a fever, which I esteemed wholly independent of the small-pox."[96]). Yet he had to go on to admit that under the pre-Suttonian method, "some of the inoculated have died under this process, even under the care of very able and experienced practitioners."[97] He qualified this admission however, by stating that "this number is so small, that, when compared with the mortality attending the natural smallpox, it is reduced almost to a cypher."[98] Given the lengthy period of preparation at this time, it is surprising that more people didn't die from infections caught previous to their inoculation, and as we have seen, even a practitioner like Barnes who was using very deep injections, was able to claim as early as 1755 that he hadn't lost one of the four hundred people inoculated by him in the Carlisle area.[99]

It was universally acknowledged however that the Suttonian innovation dramatically reduced the risks of dying from inoculation. Robert Sutton is reported to have inoculated 2,500 people between 1757 (when he first started his practice of inoculation) and 1768, without a single death[100], and the Suttons claimed in 1767 that they and their partners had inoculated fifty-five thousand people between 1760 and 1767, "of which number six only died."[101] Although it is impossible to assess this claim directly, even those with a vested interest in denying the success of inoculation did not deny the negligible mortality of the Suttonian method; for example, Jenner's statement that "a fatal instance occurred as rarely as since that [Suttonian] method was introduced."[102] This conclusion was also confirmed by independent practitioners who used the Suttonian method such as Dimsdale and Watts, who stated in 1767 that he had "been concerned in the inoculation of many hundred persons himself, and that without the misfortune of losing a single patient."[103] Daniel Sutton spread the fame of his father's technique through his spectacularly successfully mass inoculations, which received wide publicity, which was all the more impressive because it came from unsolicited independent sources. James Hallifax, vicar to the parish of Ewell in Surrey, sent the following item to the *Gentleman's Magazine* in 1766, and had it counter-signed by the local justice of the peace, a churchwarden, and two overseers of the poor:

"On the 1st July, 156 persons, chiefly inhabitants of **Ewell**, and of various ages, from six months to about sixty years, began to prepare themselves for inoculation, under the care of Mr Sutton. On the 8th of the same month they were all inoculated, most of them from a woman and her daughter in the neighbourhood . . . the eruption . . . seldom amounted to more than fifty pustules, and often fell greatly short of that number . . . Many others, animated with their success, began at different periods, to prepare themselves; insomuch, that the whole number of persons under inoculation, from the 8th of July to the 12th August, amounts to 249 persons, and Mr Sutton pronounces them all entirely out of danger from the small-pox . . . I can declare, upon my own knowledge, that from the 2nd May last (which was before Mr Sutton was known in the parish of Ewell) to this 22nd day of August, 1766, not a single person, either infant or adult, hath died, or been buried in the parish of Ewell."[104]

There are other examples of public announcements of spectacularly successful mass inoculations after the Suttonian innovation—and I suspect a systematic examination of local newspapers for the period would reveal a considerable number of these—an example being the advertisement placed by the Churchwardens and Overseers of the village of Irthlingborough, Northants in the *Northampton Mercury*:

"February 14, 1778. INOCULATED in the aforesaid Parish, by Mr Wm, Peaceful, of Twywell, in the County aforesaid, upwards of Five Hundred People; and there is not one in so large a Number, through a divine Blessing, but who has perfectly recovered."[105]

A further example was provided by Dr George Pearson, one of the first of Jenner's supporters in favouring vaccination, and a person who therefore had every reason to point up the disadvantages of inoculation where they existed:

"in the month of October (1798), 800 poor persons were inoculated for the smallpox (at Hungerford, Berkshire) without a single case of death. No exclusion was made on account of age, health, or any other circumstance, but pregnancy; one patient was eighty years of age; and many were at the breast, and in a state of toothing."[106]

These examples do not mean of course that people ceased to die from inoculation; we have seen that some inoculators still used the deep incision method late in the eighteenth century, and a number of instances of mortality from inoculation have been cited. For example, the five infants dying at Luton in 1788. But at the end of the eighteenth century, death due to inoculation was obviously becoming a rare event, and even an institution like the London Smallpox Hospital, which is known to have received cases with prior infection of smallpox, had very low inoculation mortality rates—of 5,694 people inoculated there during the years 1797-99, only nine died (0.16 per cent).[107]

Because of their willingness to act on purely empirical grounds, some of the most effective inoculators were amateurs. One of the most successful was John Williamson, who was known by his neighbours in the Shetland Islands because of his inventiveness as **Johnny Notions**. He had invented his own method of inoculation—although he may have been influenced by the Suttons—during the very severe smallpox epidemic in the Shetland Isles in 1769. His method was described in some detail by the vicar of Mid and South Yell:

"He is careful in providing the best matter, and keeps it a long time before he puts it to use—sometimes seven or eight years; and, in order to lessen its virulence, he first dries it in peat smoke, and then puts it underground, covered with camphor. Though many physicians recommend fresh matter, this self-taught practitioner finds from experience, that it always proves milder to the patient when it has lost a considerable degree of its strength. He uses no lancet in performing the operation; but, by a very small knife made by his own hands, he gently raises a very little of the outer skin of the area, so that no blood flows, then puts in a very small quantity of matter, which he immediately covers with the skin that has been thus raised. The only plaster that he uses for healing the wound is a bit of cabbage leaf. It is particularly remarkable, that there is not a single instance in his practice where the injection has not taken place, and made its appearance at the usual time. He administers no medicine during the progress of the disease, nor does he use any previous preparation . . . several thousands have been inoculated by him and he has not lost a single patient."[108]

Williamson had come near to returning the practice to its original folk simplicity, although the burial of the virus underground to lessen its effects, was quite unique to him. English amateur inoculators were just as successful as the Scottish ones, and Dr J. Forbes, although an ardent supporter of vaccination, and opponent of inoculation, had to admit that none of the many people inoculated by the amateur inoculators in the Chichester region in 1821 died. One particular amateur inoculator by the name of Pearce was especially active; he claimed "that of 10,000 persons inoculated by his father, not one died, and that his own success has been as great."[109] Forbes accepted that none of the 1,000 people inoculated by Pearce in the winter of 1821 had died.[110]

It might be thought that some of the above evidence suffers from being merely historical, and that an element of exaggeration has crept into some of the accounts of the success of inoculation. Fortunately there are recent observations on the practice of variolation (inoculation) which have been made by doctors trained and qualified up to the highest standards of modern medicine. Dr C. D. Rosenwald, who was a medical officer in Tanganika, gave the following account of variolation as it was practised in the southern province of that country in 1951:

"The material for the operation is obtained by inserting a sliver of wood into the smallpox vesicle on the skin of a person suffering from a very mild attack of smallpox. The variolous fluid is then rubbed into a superficial skin wound on the anterior or lateral aspect of the left forearm of the person whom it is wished to infect. This wound may be a cut made with a knife, or scratch or puncture made with a needle or thorn, with or without bleeding . . . There is no denying that the vast majority of cases resulting are mild. I have handled several children, examining their variolation pustules, when it has been pointed out to me that they were then actually in the active stage of smallpox. More careful examination has indeed brought to light a very small number of vesicles."[111]

An almost identical set of observations were made by Dr P. J. Imperato as a part of his work for the World Health Organisation among the Songhai in Mali, although he suggests that the effects of variolation are even milder than those found in Tanganika:

"the variolation technique used consisted of the application of vesicular fluid with either a thorn or a bird feather to a small round area of 5mm diameter on the deltoid area of the arm or the lateral aspect of the leg just below the knee. There was very little tissue destruction associated with this technique and the inoculuum was small . . . According to one infirmier who had rendered medical care to both villages during the epidemic, the sequence of events of the variolation reaction was not unlike that of a normal primary vaccinal reaction. He was aware of only two instances in which satellite lesions appeared around the edge of the variolation site . . . observations were made on 120 variolated individuals in eastern Mali. Twenty-two (18.3%) of these people subsequently developed clinical smallpox. The disease in all of these cases was mild, characterized by a rash composed of discrete lesions. There was no mortality associated with the illness."[112]

The remarkable thing about this account of Imperato's, is his belief that only 18.3 per cent of the cases developed any clinical form of smallpox; he seems to be unaware of the usual reaction to variolation—very mild forms of smallpox, with a small number of pustules—and it is likely that the pustular eruptions were so mild, that like Rosenwald's first observations, Imperato missed seeing the secondary lesions. This is very similar to the relative invisibility of the Suttonian form of inoculation; May in his account of Sutton's method for example, noted how many of the children inoculated and carried out into the streets "would escape our noticing them as under the Small-Pox, their indispositions being so very slight, and eruptions so few."[113] Like the Suttonian technique of inoculation, that used in Mali involved very superficial tissue destruction, and therefore would have achieved some of the lightest results possible (Imperato notes the existence of much severer techniques of inoculation elsewhere in Mali, involving very substantial tissue destruction—and these, like their historical counterparts, produced much severer results).[114] The wheel of this chapter has turned full circle: starting with a form of inoculation in India in 1767, remarkably similar in its technique to modern vaccination, and finishing with forms of variolation in modern Africa which are also very much like vaccination in technique and results—and all being essentially the same form of inoculation.

CHAPTER 2

The Contagiousness of Inoculation and the Process of Attenuation

As a part of his survey of variolation in Mali, Imperato interviewed a large sample of the local population about their beliefs on the contagiousness of variolation, either as witnesses or as people who had been inoculated themselves. The following Table gives a summary of the findings of the survey.[115]

Age (Years)	Total Interviewed	Variolation Reaction Can Cause Smallpox in Others					
		Yes		No		No opinion	
		Number	%	Number	%	Number	%
0-14	23	0	0	2	8.6	21	91.4
15-29	77	24	31.2	26	33.7	27	35.1
30-44	138	8	5.7	97	70.2	33	24.1
45+	209	0	0	180	86.1	29	23.9
Total	447	32	7.1	305	68.2	110	24.7

A large majority of the total sample rejected the notion that variolation could be the source of secondary contagion and spread smallpox to unprotected people, and this was particularly so among those aged thirty and above. Imperato interprets this to mean that the younger age groups have acquired a greater understanding of the correct scientific view—that variolation is a significant source of contagion—and that this is a function of their greater education. An alternative view is possible: that the younger generation has had less experience of smallpox inoculation, and that they have been persuaded through the educational process to accept the canons of conventional medical wisdom (although it should be noted that even among this younger age group, only a minority accept the contagiousness of inoculation). People above thirty would have had much greater experience of the actual effects of variolation, and it will be my contention that their view of inoculation is very substantially correct.

When inoculation was first introduced amongst medical practitioners in England in 1721, it was not thought to be contagious to those vulnerable people who came into contact with inoculated cases. Maitland had from his experience in Turkey concluded that inoculation was not infectious in the way that natural smallpox was, but was soon led to revise his opinions from his experience in England. At the beginning of October in 1721, Maitland inoculated a two-year-old girl by the name of Mary Batt, a member of a Quaker family living in Hertford; Maitland described the ensuing events as follows:

"what happen'd afterwards was, I must own, not a little surprizing to me, not having seen or observ'd any Thing like it before. The Case was in short this; Six of Mr Batt's Domestick Servants, *viz* four Man and two Maids, who all, in their Turns, were wont to hug and carress this Child whilst under the Operation, and the Pustules were out upon her, never suspecting them to be catching, nor indeed did I, were all seiz'd at once with the right natural Small Pox . . ."[116]

As there was a smallpox epidemic raging in Hertford at this time, it is possible that the servants had caught a natural form of the disease, particularly as Maitland was preparing his patients before inoculation—and he may even have infected the servants himself with respiratory virus carried from natural smallpox cases in the area. However, there is no doubt that secondary contagion did occasionally arise in England, but as we shall see later, this was almost certainly a function of the severe technique of inoculation practised by Maitland and his contemporaries.

As a result of this experience of the contagiousness of inoculation, it became a universal consensus of opinion that inoculated smallpox was merely a variant of the natural form, and as we saw in the last chapter, that the success of inoculation was due to the possibility of "managing" the disease as well as selecting a milder form of the virus with which to inoculate people. We shall see later that this was fallacious and that the severity of the smallpox case from which the virus was taken had no bearing on the outcome of inoculation itself. The contagiousness of inoculation was first questioned by Holwell in 1767 in his treatise on inoculation in Bengal, India:

"The general state of this distemper [smallpox] in the Provinces of Bengall (to which these observations are limited) is such, that for five and sometimes six years together, it passes in a manner unnoticed, from the few that are attacked with it; for the complexion of it in these years is generally so benign as to cause very little alarm; and notwithstanding the multitudes that are every year inoculated, in the usual season, it adds no malignity to the disease taken in the natural way, nor spreads the infection, as is commonly imagined in Europe."[117]

The lack of contagiousness of inoculation in India was probably partly due to the light technique of injection, and the very mild results achieved. Some inoculators began to notice a similar lack of contagiousness with the Suttonian form of inoculation, and this became a point of issue in the popular practice of the new method. Daniel Sutton believed that the "cold treatment"—

exposing patients to cool air as much as possible—was an important part of the success of his method; although he restricted his private patients to the grounds of his special inoculation house, poorer patients were returned home immediately after inoculation. May in his pamphlet on Sutton's method of inoculation, described how "we often meet with particularly children, who, for the benefit of the open air, are carried into the streets and ways, under all the different stages of Inoculation."[118] In 1765 Sutton was put on trial at Chelmsford assizes for spreading smallpox in the community at large; the Grand Jury threw out the bill, mainly on the grounds that the type of infection he produced was so light, that his patients could not become a source of secondary infection to anyone else.[119] The difficulty was, of course, that the case was difficult to prove either way, and contemporaries continued to strongly disagree about the extent of the danger of secondary infection.

This was a very important practical issue, as it affected whether patients had to be isolated from other members of the community or not; up until the Suttonian innovation, nearly all inoculated cases were isolated in special inoculation houses, and this both heavily put up the cost and restricted the number of people which could be inoculated at any one time. Daniel Sutton broke through both these constraints and was reputed to have inoculated over 100 poor people in one day, immediately returning them to their usual place of residence.[120] We shall see later that his example was almost universally copied in the country at large, but for a number of reasons was not followed in the very large towns in which about a fifth of the total population lived until the very end of the eighteenth century. Lettsom and Watkinson became concerned about the neglect of the poor in London, and attempted to remedy this situation by setting up a popular charitable institution for inoculating the poor in their own homes. This project was opposed by Dimsdale on the grounds that inoculation would spread smallpox to the unprotected population; this objection was in fact invalid on other grounds—virtually all children living in London caught smallpox by the age of seven in this period anyway—but Watkinson attempted to refute Dimsdale arguments directly on the question of secondary contagion:

"I have paid particular attention to the point in question, since the establishment of the dispensary for general inoculation; and can with truth affirm, that a single instance has not yet occurred in that charity, in which the contagion has been spread by an inoculated patient. Where the chance of spreading it has been apparently great, I have been very strict in my inquiries. In many cases the circumstances have been such, that if the apprehensions of a celebrated inoculator [Dimsdale] were well founded, the distemper must inevitably have been communicated. Some have been inoculated in narrow streets, in the midst of those who were obnoxious [vulnerable] to the smallpox, and others in little courts, where, according to the common opinion, the danger of communicating the disease was still greater. In the latter case, the patient has sometimes been kept in a little room on the ground floor, the door of which opened directly into the court, and in the day time was seldom shut. Before this door, and within a few yards of the person inoculated, a number of children have continued to play during the whole course of the disorder, and, as has been already affirmed, without receiving the infection."[121]

In addition to their own personal experience in London, Lettsom and Watkinson noted that inoculation did not appear to spread smallpox in other places. A mass inoculation took place in Ware, Herts in 1777, "and a few families in the town did not choose to submit to Inoculation with the rest of their neighbours; not one of them, however, caught the infection, although Inoculation was otherwise general ['about one hundred were inoculated']."[122] Dimsdale was sufficiently puzzled by these experiences to write to various foreign inoculators about the subject. In 1777 Professor M. W. Schwenke wrote to him from the Hague:

"I believe in England, as well as other provinces, there are some who are enemies to Inoculation, from prejudice, obstinacy and ignorance, while there are others who are deprived of its benefits by want of opportunities, or through their inability to bear the expense of it. But this does not prevent us from inoculating every year at the proper season, whether the epidemical Small Pox reigns or not; and it may be affirmed that no epidemic has ever been occasioned by this practice. The epidemical Small Pox discovers itself among us, almost regularly at certain periods, just as it did before the practice of Inoculation was introduced . . . This is certain, last year, when the epidemic which reigned with violence in our neighbourhood was expected here, I myself inoculated forty-eight persons, and a like number underwent the operation in the hands of other physicians. The inoculated persons walked, or rode out in carriages, every day (except two that were very ill) without anything like an epidemic ensuing."[123]

This letter did not change Dimsdale's views about the degree of danger of inoculation spreading smallpox. What is surprising is that Dimsdale's own experience did not lead him to modify his opinion. One writer noted the effects of inoculation in Dimsdale's county of Hertfordshire when the popular practice of the Suttonian method was introduced:

"At the introduction of that method, the subjects obnoxious to the disease were more numerous in proportion to the exempts, than they could possibly be in London at any period. Baron Dimsdale under whose direction a principle share of the practice was conducted, was not deficient in imposing such restrictions [of movement in public] on his patients as he thought necessary for public safety; but I believe these restrictions were not very scrupulously regarded. There were practitioners, whose practice was by no means inconsiderable and whose restrictions were less strenuously imposed and more frequently broken, yet few instances of infection from inoculation were heard of . . ."[124]

Some observers even pointed out that inoculation prevented the spread of smallpox; for example, Haygarth in 1781 noted that in Chester,

"Inoculation did not, as some might apprehend, spread the contagion, but appeared to produce a quite contrary effect. For in the districts, where most patients were inoculated, there remained the fewest in the natural small-pox; and in the districts where the smallest number were inoculated, the distemper was afterwards most general."[125]

This phenomena can only be explained by assuming that the inoculated cases were rarely a source of contagion, and actually reduced the number of potential carriers of the natural disease. A similar phenomena occurred in Boston, U.S.A. in 1792 during a general inoculation: 9,152 people were inoculated, yet there were only 232 cases of natural smallpox in the town, while 221 people escaped the disease altogether.[126] Inoculation in this situation checked the spread of natural smallpox, and this was not only possible through the inoculation of virtually all the vulnerable population, but also because it did not spread the disease itself (otherwise the 221 people escaping smallpox would have been infected from the 9,152 inoculated cases).

Ideally, in order to evaluate the risk of inoculation spreading smallpox, experimentation would be necessary. The only experimental evidence known to me is that accidentally supplied by Dr O'Ryan, Professor of Medicine at the College of Lyons, France, who conducted the following experiment during the latter period of the eighteenth century:

"I placed a person in the eruptive fever of the smallpox by inoculation at the distance of about half a yard from four children properly prepared; each exposure continued one hour, and was repeated daily for a fortnight, reckoning from the commencement of the fever till the pustules were become sufficiently dry: not one of the four received the infection. Two months afterwards, I inoculated three of these children, they had the distemper in a very mild manner and recovered without difficulty."[127]

O'Ryan was unaware of the difference between inoculated and natural smallpox in terms of their effect in spreading the disease, and concluded "that there is no risk of contracting it [smallpox], provided the person who is liable to the infection, keeps himself at a very little distance from patients in the smallpox, or from things which they have touched."[128] This is now known to be incorrect, for a major route of natural smallpox infection is via the respiratory tract, partly because the virus is expelled over a sufficient distance to form a significant source of contagion. The period in which the smallpox patient is infectious usually commences after the termination of the incubation period, which on average is about twelve days after the smallpox patient catches the disease.[129] In O'Ryan's experiment, the children were exposed to the inoculated patient at the time of the eruptive fever, which occurs at the end of the incubation period and therefore would be the beginning of the period of infectivity. It is therefore probable that if the inoculated patient in the experiment was highly infectious, the children would have caught the disease.

In 1791 Haygarth published a letter that he had received from the Council of Geneva, giving yet a further example of the non-contagiousness of inoculation:

"An epidemic of smallpox is of almost regular occurrence every five years, and between the epidemics it frequently happens that we have no natural smallpox whatever, little in the City or its vicinity. Inoculation began to be practised here in 1751, since when we have inoculated a very large number of children annually, and with such marked success that the deaths have not exceeded 1 in 300. Although we have often had to inoculate with pus brought from a distance at times when there was no smallpox to be found in the City, and although children so inoculated have gone freely into the streets, walks, and other public places, before, during, and after the eruption, we have never observed that they were sources of contagion, nor that they produced any intermediate epidemic, nor that they accelerated the return of the periodical epidemic."[130]

This is strong evidence for the rarity of secondary contagion from inoculation, and is very similar to that already quoted for Bengal and the Hague. Of course, in all these cases the number of susceptibles between epidemics would not be high, and would therefore reduce the risk of infection. Nevertheless, it is clear that in a place like Geneva, inoculation must have been of absolutely minimal infectivity, even during the pre-Suttonian era of the 1750's and 1760's. This evidence is the more remarkable because it refers to a place where smallpox was not present in its natural form to complicate the interpretation of events; in the absence of natural smallpox, inoculation appears to have very rarely led to secondary contagion.

However, it is almost certain that inoculation did on occasions give rise to secondary infection; ironically, the best evidence for this comes out of the history of early vaccination. I have shown in my book on Jenner's vaccine that after the initial experimental period when cowpox was used as the source of the vaccine, the main stock used by Jenner and his contemporaries became contaminated with smallpox. Nearly all the vaccine used in England and elsewhere was a strain of smallpox virus, and vaccination was in reality merely a variant of the old form of inoculation. This is an ideal situation with which to evaluate the contagiousness of inoculation, as the early vaccinators were not expecting any secondary contagion from their inoculations—vaccination was defined by Jenner as non-contagious—and the noticing of secondary contagion would be all the more impressive for not being expected. The person mainly responsible for the developing of the main stock of vaccine (the "world's lymph") was Dr William Woodville of the London Smallpox Hospital, where the contamination with smallpox had taken place; in his first report on the new vaccination he wrote:

> "One important advantage which the Cow Pox is supposed to have over the Small Pox is that the former is not a contagious disease, and not to be propagated by effluvia of persons infected with it. This is certainly true when the disorder is confined to the inoculated part, but where it produces numerous pustules on the body, the exhalations they send forth are capable of infecting others in the same manner as the Small Pox. Two instances of casual infection in this way have lately fallen under my observation . . ."[131]

Although most of Woodville's inoculations had led to relatively mild symptoms—the first 459 people to be vaccinated had an average of 78 pustules each—there were a very small minority who suffered severely, with 700 pustules or more. It is almost certain that it was these cases which gave rise to the secondary infection discussed by Woodville. The vast majority of the cases of early vaccination did not lead to secondary contagion in spite of numbers of secondary pustules, and this was partly a function of the increasingly attenuated smallpox virus being used. Only two clear examples of secondary infection from vaccinated cases have emerged to date from a study of the literature: the minor smallpox epidemic at Petworth in Sussex at the end of 1799 deriving from vaccine supplied by Dr George Pearson, and the more serious epidemic started at Marblehead near Boston in the

United States arising probably out of vaccine sent by Jenner to Benjamin Waterhouse. The vaccinated cases which started both these outbreaks of smallpox had very severe symptoms of smallpox, and it appears that there had been a spontaneous resurgence in the virulence of the virus used in the vaccinations. However, the rarity of secondary contagion from this form of smallpox inoculation is indicated by the absence of other documented examples other than the Petworth and Marblehead incidents. Undoubtedly, the more orthodox Suttonian form of inoculation did on occasions lead to secondary contagion, but the minimal degree of the nature of this contagiousness was probably accurately summarized by Haygarth when he wrote that "the danger of infection is much (perhaps thirty or fifty) less in the inoculated than the casual small-pox."[132]

Given this radical conclusion about the relative noncontagious nature of smallpox inoculation, we must raise and attempt to deal with the difficult question as to how these attenuated effects were achieved by inoculation. There is no virological or medical consensus as to how the variolators were able to achieve such successful results, and therefore the following discussion will necessarily be speculative. The first point which must be noted is that there was no one-to-one relationship between the type of virus inoculated and the severity of the results of inoculations. Initially, European inoculators believed that the success of inoculation was partly due to the mild form of virus selected for injection (i.e. virus was taken from mild clinical cases of natural smallpox), but this view was soon discredited through empirical observation. In 1749, Frewen published the following summary conclusion from his experiences:

"Experience has convinced me, that it is in reality of no consequence from what kind of Smallpox it is procured. I knew one and twenty persons inoculated, the same day, with matter taken from one who had a confluent Small-pox and died of it; yet these, notwithstanding, all had it in as favourable a way as could be wished for. And I have inoculated many more with matter of the malignant kind, without any manner of ill effect."[133]

Daniel Sutton even claimed that the results of inoculation were severer when virus was taken from a "benign" case of smallpox than when it was taken from a "malignant" one, although he produced no detailed evidence for this conclusion.[134] The irrelevancy of the severity of the disease in the person from whom the virus was taken for inoculation was further confirmed by Mudge in his dissertation on inoculation published in 1777:

"Several patients have been inoculated from a confluent smallpox, which have proved mortal to its own subject, and yet have had the disorder in a very favourable way. Others have been inoculated from malignant sorts with equal success; nay, which is still more, we are told by Chandler in his essay, that in inoculating hospitals, persons have been safely infected with matter which has been taken off after the death of the patient. These, and other instances which must have occurred to men of business in this way, plainly shew that the **benignity** of the infecting matter has very little share in the wonderful effects of inoculation."[135]

This conclusion had become generally accepted by the end of the eighteenth century and Woodville summarized the consensus of opinion when he wrote in 1797 that it does not "signify whether the matter is taken from a mild kind or from the more virulent sort."[136]

    This conclusion may have come to affect the medical view about the relationship between intrinsic virulence and clinical severity of natural smallpox. Generally, it has been the view of microbiologists and virologists until very recently, that the clinical severity of smallpox was in the main not a function of its intrinsic virulence. The only exception to this view was the distinction between variola major and variola minor, the former being much more virulent than the latter. In the last few years however, evidence has begun to accumulate to suggest that this view is mistaken. Marennikova and Shafikova have carried out research involving the comparative study of the properties of various variola virus strains taken from patients with varying clinical severity of the disease; they found that "the virus strains isolated from patients suffering from haemorrhagic forms of smallpox were usually more pathogenic for chick embryos than those isolated from other forms of the disease."[137] The degree of statistical significance of these findings is not however very great and they go against the mainstream conclusions of modern virological research, which tend to show little correlation between clinical severity of individual cases of smallpox and laboratory measures of intrinsic virulence. On the other hand, it has now been established that the severity of particular strains of smallpox virus within specific geographical areas are significantly correlated with laboratory measures of virulence. Shafikova and Marennikova found a relationship between fourteen strains isolated from patients with different severities of smallpox, and pathogenicity for suckling and irradiated adult white mice inoculated intracerebrally and intranasally.[138] Also, work carried out in conjunction with the W.H.O. smallpox eradication campaign involving the laboratory study of 200 strains of virus from all parts of the world, has tended to show quite distinct geographical patterns of pathogenicity, suggesting a number of specific regional viruses. Dumbell and Huq have questioned the validity of the distinction between variola

major and variola minor and have concluded that "recent observations during the smallpox eradication campaign fit in better
with the idea of a spectrum of variola viruses of differing pathogenicity, ranging from a minimum in Brazil to a maximum in
Bangladesh."[139] This conclusion is consistent with the fact that
the pathogenicity of smallpox is known to have varied enor-
mously within a particular region over long periods of time; for
example, as we shall see later, the case-fatality of smallpox was
of the order of five per cent in England at the end of the sixteenth
century, and rose to over forty per cent by the middle of the
nineteenth century.

A related finding of recent research which has a direct
bearing on the explanation of the very mild results achieved by
variolation, has come out of the work of Sarkar and his colleagues in India. Sarker et. al. studied the relationship between
the clinical severity of smallpox and the excretion of virus in the
throat and urine and found that "clinically more severe (haemorrhagic and confluent) cases excrete more virus than less severe
(discrete) cases and the period of excretion is longer in the first
two groups than in the last."[140] This conclusion applies to variations of clinical severity within one particular strain of virus,
and again is not highly statistically significant and would tend
to go against the mainstream of virological research. The correlation between clinical severity and period of infectivity does
however probably apply to different strains of smallpox virus
in specific geographical regions, for as Dixon has noted, with
milder forms of smallpox

"the period of infectivity is exceedingly short, only lasting a
few hours, and the quantity of virus small, and if this occurs
at night this patient is quite likely to miss infecting any
contacts, even those living in the same house. This has been
noticed particularly in outbreaks of variola minor, where . . .
the low degree of infectivity has been frequently commented
upon."[141]

However, there is obviously no simple one-to-one relationship
between clinical severity and infectiousness; the historical literature provides abundant examples of a single strain being introduced into a community with a complete spectrum of severity of
symptomology resulting. This means that an apparently mild
case of smallpox may in fact be the manifestation of a virologi-
cally virulent strain, with a highly infectious nature. If however
inoculation produced a fundamental attenuation of the smallpox
virus—as would appear to be the case—this would lead to a radically diminished power of infectivity.

We have now reached the point where we must consider
the central question as to how inoculation brought about such a
radical attenuation of symptomology. The first hypothesis which

comes to mind is the route by which the virus is introduced into the body; in natural smallpox infection, the virus enters via the respiratory tract, while in inoculation as practised in Europe, it was always introduced via the skin. There is one major insurmountable objection to this hypothesis, at least in its simplest form as put forward above: in China, Persia and elsewhere, the virus was introduced by inoculation through the nasal passage, presumably entering the respiratory tract in the usual way; yet the results appear to have been as successful with this method of inoculation as with the more usual mode via the skin. Although no scholarly study of Chinese inoculation has ever been published, there is sufficient evidence to come to certain tentative conclusions. It seems to have been a long-standing practice, probably extending over hundreds of years. One of the most detailed accounts of Chinese inoculation was published by Dr W. W. Peter at the end of the nineteenth century:

"One (method of inoculating) is . . . plugging the nostrils with cotton previously saturated with a mixture of water and pustular-crustaceous matter taken from the eruption of a smallpox patient. Another is to blow finely crushed fresh scabs into the nose through a bamboo pipe. It may also be done by introducing the smallpox matter through a puncture, an incision or an abraded surface of the skin . . . The crop is less profuse than in ordinary smallpox and limited to about two hundred points . . . About one in five hundred die."[142]

Most of the other descriptions of Chinese inoculation available in the English literature confirm Peter's account,[143] although at least one report indicated that the operation was not always as predictably safe as suggested by him.[144] The most frequent method of inoculation seems to have been the blowing of dried scab powder up the patient's nose, which appears to have been as successful as the more usual method of injection via the skin. Given the great variety of routes of inoculation employed by the variolators, it would seem that the route of inoculation is not crucial in the explanation of the success of variolation.

Wheelock has recently put forward an ingenious hypothesis for the relative benignity of inoculated smallpox: that when variolators took matter from a smallpox pustule or crust, they were also taking interferon, which is known to both appear in dermal crusts of vaccinated cases, and be an effective antiviral agent.[145] There are however a number of fairly critical objections to this hypothesis: interferon was only found in four out of five crusts, which would lead to a much higher failure rate than experienced in inoculation, and it probably is not as stable as would be required by some of the historical evidence, i.e. it is unlikely to have been able to survive the seven to eight years burial underground as practised in John Williamson's highly successful mode of inoculation. The most important objection however to Wheelock's hypothesis is that it cannot account for a number of observations made on the process of attenuation through arm-to-arm inoculation, or the role of the depth of the injection in bringing about milder symptomology as discussed in the first chapter.

In my book on Jenner's vaccine, I have produced a great deal of evidence to show that the smallpox virus used in Woodville's lymph was gradually attenuated through arm-to-arm inoculation, always selecting virus from a previous site of injection. I argued that this process of attenuation was achieved through the natural selection of "cold variants" that were particularly adaptable to the cooler areas of the skin surface than the more virulent strains of virus. There are good reasons to believe that a similar argument can be applied to the explanation of the benignity of more conventional forms of variolation. We have seen in the previous chapter how the depth of the injection was so important to the outcome of inoculation, and it can be hypothesized that the temperature gradient between the skin's surface and the inner body areas is the critical variable in explaining this fact. More specifically, the lighter injections of the sort practised by the Suttons would implant the virus in the epidermis, whereas the heavier inoculations practised by the early European inoculators would push the virus through the dermis into—in many cases—the blood stream. Timoni described how many of these heavy inoculations either failed altogether or brought about a very severe reaction. Although these diametrically opposed responses would appear to be paradoxical, they do in fact fit what one would expect from a number of experimental observations, as we shall now see.

Daniel Sutton conducted a series of trial inoculations, which were summarized by him in his book on inoculation in 1796:

"I have . . . repeatedly tried to communicate the disease, by conveying considerable quantities of active virus into the stomach, in the form of pills, but never with effect; both cool and typical clysters of water, strongly impregnated with the contents of many ripe and unripe pustules, have likewise been administered; this way too, I have always failed of communicating the disease."[146]

In addition to these experiments, he attempted to inoculate a number of people with very deep skin injections, again without success.[147] Smallpox virus is known to be highly temperature-sensitive, and the prediliction of the virus for the skin surface is probably the result of its ceiling temperature. Variola major will not grow on the chorio-allantois above 38.5°C or variola minor

37.9°C, whereas the body temperature reaches 39.4°C and above during the second day and onwards of the illness of smallpox[148]— suggesting that fever is a defensive response of the body against such viral attacks. As Downie has noted, "the onset of fever in smallpox might limit growth in the internal organs while permitting such growth in the skin and in mucous membranes of the mouth and upper respiratory tract, where temperatures may be a degree or two less."[149] Recent unpublished research by Dumbell however, indicates that smallpox virus can grow at higher temperatures in human than in chick cells, and these ceiling temperatures are, therefore, probably not so critical as they appear from the published evidence. Similarly although earlier work suggested a correlation between virulence and ceiling temperature for many of the pox viruses,[150] recent and unpublished work also by Dumbell indicates little association between the case-fatality rate of a particular strain of smallpox virus and laboratory measures of ceiling temperature. There is however one naturally occurring form of "cold" smallpox virus—the strain previously identified as variola minor. There is also experimental evidence to suggest that temperature can be critical in bringing about changes in the virulence in some of the pox viruses. Kirn and Braunwald produced a cold variant of vaccinia by growing the virus at regularly decreasing temperatures, losing completely "its virulence in mice by the intracerebral route" and its intradermal infectivity in rabbits was 41 times weaker than the wild virus.[151] Similarly, Baxby found a correlation between the pathogenicity of seven smallpox vaccines for human beings and their capacity to grow at elevated temperatures on the chick chorioallantois.[152] Relevant to the present argument is the work of Dumbell, Bedson and Nizamuddin, who have successfully produced a thermo-efficient strain of variola major virus. Two strains of virus were grown at increasing temperatures through serial passage in the chick choriallantois, and both became genetically stable viruses capable of greater growth at higher temperatures; one of them—which had been grown at regularly increasing temperatures without a pass at a lower temperature—was also less capable of growth at the lower temperature.[153]

Bringing together all these observations, we may hypothesize that the deep injections of the early inoculators partly failed because they were putting virus directly into the blood stream, the temperature of which was higher than that in the epidermis. However, at the same time, a process of natural selection can be seen as to have been at work, with only thermo-efficient strains of virus being able to grow in the higher temperatures of the blood—thus the paradoxical finding described by Timoni, that either there was no reaction to the deep injection, or there was a very pathogenic one. Virus found in skin lesions is likely to be a "colder variant" of that found in the blood;

more thermo-efficient viruses would simply not be able to survive the cooler temperatures at the skin's surface. Thus when inoculators took virus from skin lesions they would be selecting a form of cold variant—human selection of virus which had been naturally selected on grounds of temperature. Although this hypothesis cannot be proven with the evidence which is at present available, it has the merit of being consistent with both the historical and modern virological literature—and linking: (i) findings about the attenuation of smallpox virus through arm-to-arm inoculation in early vaccination; (ii) the importance of the depth of injection in the success of inoculation; and (iii) the overall explanation of the benignity of inoculated smallpox compared to the natural form of the disease.

It should be stressed however that the above is highly speculative and in no way crucial to the overall argument. Much recent evidence would appear to go against any simple "cold variant" hypothesis, and it is possible that alternative virological explanations—for example, that the inoculation of a large amount of virus would bring about attenuation through propagating "defective" viruses—will turn out to be more plausible. Whatever the ultimate virological explanation, it is clear that an identical virus can be made to specialize in particular organ sites, dramatically limiting its capacity to propagate outside of its zone of specialization. Ledingham and McClean found as long ago as 1928 that vaccinia virus propagated in the rabbit dermis through serial passage, led to enhanced potency of the virus for the dermis, but a "loss of propagating power on scarification surfaces"[154], i.e. virus adapted to grow in the dermis, lost its capacity to grow effectively on the skin surface. Smallpox virus selected from the skin surface for purposes of inoculation, is likely to have been relatively specialized for growth in the skin, with only limited capacity for generalisation throughout the body. A similar consideration applies to the attenuation of smallpox virus using arm-to-arm inoculation in the early practice of vaccination, and this is related to inoculation having been merely a slightly less attenuated form of injection than early vaccination. Although inoculation spread secondary infection on very rare occasions, this was more than counter-balanced by the longer period of immunity produced through the larger and more effective amount of antibody (inoculation protected in the vast majority of cases for life). Also, ironically the belief that inoculated smallpox was as contagious as the natural form of the disease, led many communities to adopt the practice of general inoculation—the inoculation of all vulnerable members of a community at one point in time. But this, and other aspects of the history of inoculation, will be dealt with in the following chapters.

CHAPTER 3

The Early Practice of Inoculation and Factors in its Retardation

In April 1721 Lady Mary Wortley Montagu had her daughter inoculated in London, and from this date onwards inoculation came into fashion amongst the aristocracy and gentry, particularly after Princess Caroline had her two daughters Amelia and Caroline inoculated in April 1722. According to the inoculation censuses conducted by Jurin and Scheuchzer during the 1720s, there were 897 inoculations in Britain, America and Hanover during the eight years 1721-28.[155] After 1728 no attempt was made to count the number of inoculations, which led Creighton to conclude that:

"for the next ten or twelve years they were of no account. The southern counties led the revival in the fifth decade of the century, so that before long some two thousand had been inoculated in Surrey, Kent, Sussex and Hampshire."[156]

This conclusion has been questioned by Miller who has argued that at no time did inoculation cease to be practised, and quoted the examples of inoculations taking place in Haverford West, Pembrokeshire in 1732, in Bury and Dumfries, Scotland during 1733, and in Ireland in 1734.[157] However, she also points out that "the number of publications on the subject declined, so that during the 1730s one finds only a few pamphlets and occasional journal articles."[158]

The decline of inoculation was noted by the Rev. J. Hough who wrote in 1737 that "the method loses ground, even in this country."[159] Charles Deering, a medical practitioner in Nottingham, argued in a treatise on smallpox written in 1737 that "all who are inoculating do well, yet such is the way of thinking amongst the Generality of Man . . . that not one in five thousand either submits or is submitted to that Operation."[160] Thus, although Deering indicates that inoculation was not very popular, he does suggest that it was still being practised in 1737. This conclusion is confirmed by an entry in the diary of John Hervey, First Earl of Bristol: "on new years day (1736/37) arriv'd at London, with Miss Betty Hervey to be inoculated."[161] It was necessary for Hervey to travel to London to obtain inoculation, which suggests that it must have been rarely practised in the countryside.

Whatever the changes in the amount of inoculation during 1721-40, contemporaries were unanimous on the insignificance of the practice at any time during this period. Jurin explained in 1724 why the practice was not more popular: "People do not easily come into a practice, in which they appreciate any hazard, unless they are frightened into it by a greater danger."[162] We shall see later that the fear of catching natural smallpox (particularly during epidemics) was invariably a necessary stimulant to the practice of popular inoculation. The psychology of this attitude is not difficult to understand, for a remote risk, however dangerous, is often preferable to an immediate one. This fact was noted by the Rev. J. Hough in 1737 when attempting to explain why inoculation was losing ground:

"for parents are tender and fearful, not without hope their children may escape this disease, or have it favourably, whereas, in the way of art, should it prove fatal, they could never forgive themselves: for this reason, nobody dares to advise in the case."[163]

Such an attitude could flourish only where there was a known risk of dying from inoculation, and as we have earlier seen the practice of inoculation was fairly dangerous during the period under discussion.

Another important factor in the retardation of the spread of inoculation was its very high cost during the early period. One gentleman wrote the following entry into his diary in 1743:

"Memorandum the 17th of January this year, my son and Miss Molly Tregonwell were both inoculated by Mr Goldwyer, Surgeon of Blandford, whose pay for the said inoculation was 20 guineas."[164]

Inoculation was so expensive at this time because of the lengthy period of preparation and after-treatment in special isolation houses, along with the complicated procedures of blood-letting and purging, as well as the special medicines prescribed by attendant physicians. The 10 guineas per person would have included board and lodging during the five or six week period "necessary" for the whole operation. The above example was not untypical of the period, as is seen in the accounts of the Bristol Infirmary where £623 was paid for the inoculation of 78 people in 1743.[165] Inoculation was to be had for a cheaper rate under special circumstances, such as the inoculation of the poor. One gentleman wrote in 1750 that:

"Several years ago a noble person near Guildford in Surrey, observing the terror of the country people, on account of the small-pox, allowed Mr Howard a skilful surgeon of that place, the sum of 40s. for every one that he should inoculate and attend."[166]

This price differential between the rich and the poor was maintained throughout the whole of the eighteenth century, although the absolute level of prices was very radically reduced. The price of inoculation during the period 1721-50 was obviously too high for the great bulk of the population, and in 1752 one writer observed that:

> "before it can come into general use, it must be done in a less expensive way . . . The poor in general are absolutely cut off from all share in it . . . And not only the very poor people, but multitudes of others, many farmers and tradesmen, cannot be at the expence of so much a head for their whole family, as it is at present demanded, merely for the operation of inoculating, besides the other additional charges which must necessarily accrue."[167]

And the high price of inoculation continued to deter people from undergoing the operation as late as 1760, for when a smallpox epidemic struck the Shetland Islands in 1760, "owing to the high fee (two or three guineas) of the operator, only ten or twelve persons availed themselves of it."[168]

A less important factor retarding the spread of inoculation was the opposition due to religious opinion. In 1724 W. Beeston wrote a letter on the subject from Ipswich:

> "The practice of Inoculation in this Town, has so inflamed the angry passions, and stirred up the bitter Zeale of the bigotted high Churchmen, and Dissentors, to such a Degree: that they Sentence to Damnation, all that are in any way Concerned in it. They say the practice is Heathenish, and Diabolicall, it is distrusting Providence, and taking the Power out of God's hand, it will draw down Divine Judgments . . ."[169]

The most notorious religious opposition came from the Rev. Edmund Massey, who preached on "The Dangerous and Sinful Practice of Inoculation" from the pulpit of the parish church of St. Andrews, Holborn (London) on July 8th, 1722.[170] More important than formal religious opposition though, was popular prejudice against inoculation which although couched in religious terms, was really a reflection of emotional attitudes to death, and the anxiety about incurring deliberate risks for a future remote gain. Dr John Andrew illustrated this from his experience in the Exeter area:

> "The chief Argument urged by foolishly fond or superstitious Parents, against this Practice, is, that it brings a Distemper upon their Children, which they might never have, and that if any one of them should die, they should never forgive themselves, on Account of their having (as they term it) presumptuously tempted Providence."[171]

Partly as a result of these prejudices, Andrew was forced at the beginning of the 1740s to practise inoculation "in the Dark, visiting my Patients only by Night."[172]

However, the major reason why Andrew was forced to practice inoculation under cover of darkness, was probably fear by the general population that his inoculations would spread smallpox within the community. A similar experience to his took place soon after the London Smallpox Hospital was set up in 1746, and patients who had been inoculated, "on leaving the hospital were often abused and insulted in the street, so that they were not suffered to depart until the darkness of the night enabled them to do so without being observed."[173] The Fear of inoculation spreading smallpox sometimes led to drastic action on the part of the local population, particularly when there was no natural smallpox in the area:

"Sutton and Bond, inoculators, having opened a house near Peterborough, the mob rose, to prevent, as they said, the spreading of infection, by introducing a distemper that was not then in that neighbourhood, and threatened to pull down the house, which they effected next day, after an obstinate resistance, in which several were wounded, and the undertakers obliged to decamp."[174]

Hostility to inoculation on these grounds was particularly strong in market towns, where there was great anxiety that a whiff of smallpox would ruin local trade. This was reflected in innumerable entries in local newspapers; for example, on May 12, 1762 the following announcement appeared in a Colchester paper:

"The Practice of bringing people out of the country into this town to be inoculated for the Small-pox being very prejudicial to the town in many respects, but especially to the Trade thereof, and as by this practice the distemper may be continued much longer in the town than it otherwise would, in all probability, it is thought proper by some of the principal inhabitants and traders in the town, that this public notice should be given that they are determined to prosecute any person or persons whomsoever, that shall hereafter bring into this town, or who shall receive into their houses in the town as lodgers, any person for that purpose, with the utmost severity that the law will permit . . ."[175]

The announcement went on to state that it had no objection to the practice of inoculation, as long as it was conducted in houses well isolated from the town. The fear of the townsmen that inoculation would spread natural smallpox was, of course, based on the contemporary assumption that it was just a milder

form of smallpox, which was thought to be as dangerous as the
most virulent form of smallpox.

There was also popular opposition to inoculation on
medical grounds, although like the belief in the highly contagiousness nature of the operation, it was not always based
on an objective foundation. D. Hartley, listed in a pamphlet
published in 1733, the following medical objections made by the
general population:

> "We are not certain that Inoculation is a Security from hav-
> ing the Distemper again . . . inoculated **Small Pox** often
> leaves bad Consequences, as Consumptions, Boils, and
> Blotches, weak Eyes, etc . . . [and] may communicate other
> Distempers."[176]

Hartley could not refrain from pointing out, "that the natural
Small Pox is apt to leave the same Sort of ill Consequences, is
known to everyone",[177] only to a much greater degree. The medical profession itself was by no means unanimous in the earlier
period in favour of inoculation; as late as 1747, Mead could
write that inoculation "has drawn our physicians into parties,
some approving, and others disapproving this new practice."[178]

By far the most important factor in the removal of
checks on the spread of inoculation was the reduction of mortality from the operation due to the improvements of technique,
as was shown by the very rapid spread of inoculation after the
innovations made by the Sutton family. The latter point is illustrated by contemporary descriptions of the effect of the successful Suttonian method:

> "it is natural to suppose that the great success attending, and
> emoluments arising from the Suttonian art, may induce
> many to become imitators of their method of inoculation.
> And in fact this is so much the case, that in every county in
> England you meet with the advertisements of these pre-
> tenders and itinerants . . . Some of them as before observed,
> advertise that they inoculate according to the **new method**;
> others according to the **Suttonian method**; while others have
> the modesty to deck their imposition with the style of,
> 'The Suttonian art improved'."[179]

In fact, as we will see later in much greater detail, the
Suttonian method was the beginning of the really popular practice of inoculation. In order for this to be possible, it was necessary for the price of inoculation to be radically reduced from
what it was during the earlier period. This was carried out by
the Suttons who introduced differential prices acording to the
type of inoculation and the financial circumstances of their
patients. The following advertisement was placed in the *Norwich
Mercury* on the 25th January, 1777:

"Messrs. Sutton and Son respectfully inform the public that they continue to inoculate for the small-pox at their house in Framingham, near Norwich, on the most reasonable terms. The greatest respect being had to various circumstances of the patients different accommodations are provided from two guineas and a half to ten and upwards. General terms, four guineas. The small-pox being at present very rife not only in Norwich, but in most parts of the county of Norfolk, Messrs. Suttons continue as usual to inoculate parties at their own houses on terms agreeable to circumstances from half a guinea upwards. Servants and the poor in general (not less than eight in number) at five shillings and threepence . . . The officer of any parish, by applying to Messrs. Suttons, may have their poor inoculated gratis."[180]

This type of price discrimination became the most frequent method by which the professional inoculators maximized both numbers inoculated and profit. Not all medical practitioners were concerned about profit, as is shown by an entry which appeared in the *Northampton Mercury*:

"To the Poor of Northampton. As the Small-Pox now prevails on the Town, and many Persons wish to have their Children Inoculated, but are deprived of this Advantage by their Inability to defray the Expence. Dr Hardy informs all Persons of this Description, that on their producing to him a Certificate signed by the Minister or Churchwarden of their respective Parishes, that their circumstances are such as must render the Expence inconvenient, He will prepare, inoculate, and atend them through the disease, Gratis."[181]

That this was not an isolated humanitarian charitable gesture is shown by the following description of other charitable inoculations:

"Such being the salutory effects of inoculation . . . To this benevolent and public spirited purpose several excellent charitable institutions, both in London and in the country, are entirely devoted; with this view, also, many opulent individuals have been at great pains to introduce it among their tenants, work people; and the (medical) Faculty have shown such a laudable readiness to contribute the utmost of their assistance to the establishment of the practice, that the poor may, almost every where, have their children inoculated gratis; and have even, in some cases, been assisted with money, clothes, medicines, etc. during the course of the disease."[182]

This type of charitable inoculation occurred as early as the 1740s when a local gentleman paid the 40 shillings per head for some of the poor in the Guildford area. However, a much more important form of inoculation was that provided by parish authorities for their "poor". The first record we have of a mass inoculation being paid for by the overseers of the poor is that which took place in 1756 when a large number of the parish poor were inoculated during the smallpox epidemic at Wootten-under-Edge, a market town in Gloucestershire.[183] As the Webbs have pointed out, the poor were defined so as to include most of the wage-earning population for purposes of medical relief.[184] This is illustrated by the general inoculation which took place in Northwold, Norfolk in 1788:

> "It was therefore resolved that a general innoculation of such uninfected persons should take place and as the Major part of such persons were unabel to Defray the necessary Expence of innoculating themselves and their families, it was purposed that the Churchwardens should be Impowered by a future meeting to Borrow a sum, not exceeding thirty pounds, free from the payment of Interest on the Credit of the town Estate, which was Given among other purposes for Charitabel Uses."[185]

A total of 300 people were inoculated, 226 of which were "inoculated on the Parish Charge". The remaining 74 were paid for by the heads of families who could afford to pay for their own inoculations; according to a list of these 25 heads of families, most of them were farmers and artisans—presumably master artisans trading on their own account.[186] The actual cost of inoculation to the parish and the heads of families was 2 shillings per person.

The price of inoculating the poor was relatively low as early as 1758 when the parish of Beaminster, Dorset paid 5 shillings per head for 27 of its inhabitants.[187] Similarly, the parish of Rye, Sussex paid the local surgeon Frewer two shillings and sixpence per head for inoculating "329 poor persons" in 1767— a total sum of £41. 2s. 6d.[188] Most students of overseer of the poor accounts have noted the very large sums of money spent on mass and general inoculations.[189] One of the reasons why parishes were prepared to incur such heavy expenditure was the very heavy alternative cost of having to nurse and sometimes bury smallpox cases. Perhaps an extreme example of this is to be found at Thaxted, Essex in 1717, when it cost the parish £6. 17s. 3d. to feed and nurse a family, "Widow Mallie's having the smallpox".[190] Contemporaries were very aware of the economic advantages of inoculation; the Rev. Stuart described how before the successful general inoculation of 1788, smallpox had cost the parish a great deal, both directly and indirectly:

> "For nine years that I have had the living of Luton, the average number of small-pox patients is 25. These, at the

lowest computation, stand the parish at two guineas each, exclusive of medical assistance. The disease is so apprehended in the country, that the nurses require double pay; and both they and the patients are confined in an airinghouse several weeks after the recovery . . . But, alas! these fifty guineas are but a small part of the real charge and inconvenience produced by this dreadful malady. Its almost constant effect is a permanent augmentation of the parish expenditure. If a labourer dies, his family must be supported. If a mother is lost, the children must be removed to a workhouse, as their father cannot spare time for employments that are merely domestic."[191]

As inoculation of the parish poor cost "not more than two shillings", Stuart advocated that a "plan of annual inoculations take place."[192] That this kind of heavy parish expenditure on smallpox was typical, is indicated by the study of parish poor accounts; according to E. G. Thomas who has analyzed the Essex accounts:

"smallpox was the greatest scourge with which the overseer had to contend, and it was, at the same time, the severest drain on the poor rate entailing expensive nursing charges and costs attendant on the isolation of the victims. References are made to the disease in almost every account book."[193]

This type of expenditure was obviously an incentive to parish authorities to inoculate their poor, at least when it had become sufficiently cheap by the 1750s. The price of inoculation paid for by the parish was rarely greater than 5 shillings or less than 2 shillings during the latter half of the eighteenth century.

Although the price of inoculation was relatively low during this period, many parishes were reluctant to pay for the inoculation of their poor. Dimsdale described in 1776 the variations from parish to parish in Hertfordshire:

"in the county of Hertford, there have been two methods of public or general inoculation; one to inoculate, at a low price, as many inhabitants of any small town or village, as could be persuaded to submit to it, and at the same time were able to pay, refusing all those who had it not in their power to procure the money demanded. The other method has been, where the inhabitants of a town, or a district, of all denominations, have agreed to be inoculated at the same time, the parish officers or some neighbouring charitably disposed persons, having first promised to defray the expense, and provide subsistence for such of the poor, as are unable to pay for themselves."[194]

The reason for the reluctance of some parishes to pay for the inoculation of their poor was discussed by Dimsdale, and the following lengthy quotation reveals in a humorously macabre fashion the basic attitude of some parish authorities towards the whole question:

"But such is the obstinacy of some parishes, and the parsimony of others, that it is impossible for the poor who are desirous of being inoculated, to persuade them to advance the small sum that would be necessary to defray the expense; and they are therefore obliged to wait the event of the natural disease, while the principal inhabitants are securing their own families by Inoculation. Another unjustifiable piece of frugality that deserves attention and to be remedied is, that in many places where the whole number of poor have been inoculated at the expence of the parish, illiterate fellows, totally unacquainted with diseases or remedies, have been employed on account of cheapness only, when at the same time the families of the wealthy have been under the care of medical gentlemen of good reputations . . . The inhabitants of a certain parish had a meeting to agree on inoculating all the poor, some medical gentlemen in the neighbourhood offered to undertake the business at a very low price; but as cheapness was the only object of consideration, the parish was about to agree with a blacksmith at eighteen pence a head, when one of the most frugal stated this objection: 'It is very probable that under this man's care we may have some die, and the expence of their burial may cost the parish so much, that it might as well agree with a better man.' This objection was thus removed by the smith: 'Come, I'll tell you what I'll do with you—Give me half a crown a head, and them that die I will carry to the Churchyard without putting the parish to any further expence.' "[195]

A very similar and macabrely humorous experience occurred to Edward Jenner in 1800; he had offered to gratuitously vaccinate the poor of a neighbouring parish to Cheltenham, which was refused until:

"The cost of coffins for those who were cut off by smallpox proved burdensome to the parish; the churchwardens, therefore, moved by this argument effectually exerted their authority and compelled the people to avail themselves of Dr Jenner's kind offer."[196]

Economic considerations were obviously of primary importance in determining the attitudes of parish authorities towards the inoculation of the poor. Such a strict parsimonious attitude illustrated in the above accounts inevitably led to the realisation that it was cheaper to inoculate the poor than to nurse, feed, isolate and sometimes bury them after they had caught natural smallpox. I have already indicated the high cost of such a parish responsibility, which may be further illustrated by the expenditure of the parish of Castle Combe, Wiltshire in 1758 as the result of a smallpox epidemic: the total expenditure on the poor was £141, which was more than double the usual average.[197] It paid such a parish to inoculate its poor rather than pay the expenses associated with a natural epidemic—the parish could have inoculated 560 people for the sum of £70, assuming that each inoculation cost two shillings and sixpence per head, and it is unlikely that the number needing inoculation was as high as 560. Not all poor would have to be paid for by the parish, as sometimes employers paid for the inoculation of their servants, in order to minimize the danger to their own families (advertisements requiring servants to have been inoculated before they could be employed, were common throughout the eighteenth century).

Dimsdale in his account of inoculation in Hertfordshire mentioned large numbers of amateur inoculators who were practising during the period (1776). Although he adopted a very critical attitude towards them, he had to admit:

"that many instances can be produced, where whole parishes of poor have been inoculated, and have succeeded very well, under the care of persons who were totally unacquainted with medicine. I will not here dispute the truth of this assertion."[198]

The amateur inoculators were important in both reducing the price of inoculation and making it available to that section of the population who could not obtain it through their parish. In fact from the very beginning of the practice of inoculation in England in the 1720s, it was carried out by people outside the medical profession; some amateurs were practising as itinerant inoculators by the early 1760s, for Dr Thomas Glass described at the end of 1766 how "four or five years since I was desired to visit a Girl, who had been inoculated, with thirteen or fourteen other persons, at a farm-house in the neighbourhood of Honiton [in Devon], by an itinerant Operator."[199] The practice of inoculation by amateurs seems to have accelerated with the simplification of method and technique, particularly that associated with the Suttonian innovation; for example, the resident surgeon of the Foundling Hospital in London wrote in 1768:

"Very great success has likewise attended inoculation in many parts of this kingdom: even though it has of late descended into very illiterate hands (a livery servant, belonging to a friend of the author's left his master's service, not a great while since, to practice inoculation)."[200]

This was the time when the success of the Sutton family led to the imitations by "pretenders and itinerants" described by Houlton.

Although amateurs practised inoculation cheaper than the professionals, they were still concerned with the profitability of the practice, and even the blacksmith in the Hertfordshire parish involved in the dispute over costs was asking for a minimum of one shilling and sixpence per head. It is possible that these amateur inoculators made a smaller charge to the ordinary poor when they had to pay for themselves, although there is no evidence on this. One way of having inoculation without paying for it was mentioned by William Buchan in the 1769 edition of his *Domestic Medicine*:

> "Should all other methods fail, we would recommend it to parents to perform the operation themselves . . . I have known many instances even of mothers performing the operation."[201]

As late as 1824, a member of the medical profession could report from Canterbury that "the most zealous inoculators were females—often the parents themselves—frequently officious friends . . ."[202], and four years earlier, Cross had reported that of the many people operating in East Anglia, "the greatest inoculators were the parents of poor children, farriers, blacksmiths, tailors, shoemakers, and old women."[203] Clearly, many parents had taken Buchan's advice, particularly amongst the poor, although obviously other kinds of amateur inoculators flourished well into the 19th century.

The opposition to inoculation on religious grounds seems to have diminished relatively rapidly. In 1753 a Chelmsford surgeon noted:

> "As to religious objections they are almost given up as 'tis high time they should (except amongst a few bigots indeed) . . . the learned bishop of Worcester's sermons one wou'd think sufficient to remove all kind of objections, religious as well as other, with all reasonable people."[204]

This diminution of religious opposition to inoculation was not confined to the educated, for the same Chelmsford surgeon observed:

> "This universal good is inoculation, and notwithstanding envy has laid such batteries against it, yet happy for this kingdom it gains ground daily; the lower class of people coming into it very fast in these parts."[205]

Opposition to inoculation on religious grounds never entirely disappeared at any time during the eighteenth century; for example, William Buchan claimed in 1769 that "the first step

towards rendering the practice universal must be to remove the
religious prejudices against it."[206] However, religious opposition
was not strong enough in itself to retard the spread of inoculation, as is illustrated in the following account of conflict between a Congregational Pastor and his Hitchin, Herts. congregation:

"It was in 1771, a year when the smallpox raged. They were
burying townsmen that summer by the score, and throughout the county also, insomuch that Dimsdale, the famous
inoculator, opened an 'inoculating house' at Hertford under
his own supervision. Foreseeing what was going to happen,
Hickman warned his people that 'inoculation was a kind
of presuming upon Providence', and that he should refuse
to pray for anyone who had recourse to it. In terror for
their lives, the richer brethren resolved to trust to the practice of a clever Quaker inoculator [Dimsdale] rather than
to the preaching of their solid Independent pastor. They
remembered that his wife had died of the small-pox, in
spite of all his prayers, only two years before. They made
the journey to Hertford and were saved. The poorer members, who could not afford to go to Hertford, had perforce
to stay at home and trust in Providence, and several of them
died. Unfortunately for Hickman it was the richer sort he
had to look to for his stipend, and they were not minded to
pay for a minister who would not pray for them. There was
nothing for it, therefore, but [for Hickman] to shut down
his school and look for better treatment in another part of
the country."[207]

It was because the congregation were in "terror of their lives"
that they dispensed with the services of their minister, along
with his traditional religious attitudes. The most effective demonstration of the decline of religious opposition to inoculation is
found in the actual proportions of populations inoculated by
the end of the eighteenth century—a topic to be treated at
length in the next chapter. Most of the evidence for the persistence of religious opposition to inoculation concerns large
towns; for example, Turner writing about Newcastle in 1792
noted:

"there still subsists, especially amongst the lower classes, a
great and general prejudice against the practice of inoculation; and some of the most popular grounds of this prejudice have obtained a degree of credit by claiming to be
found in religion."[208]

Edinburgh that
Similarly, one medical observer noted in 1786 with reference to

"although among the higher ranks inoculation is now become universal, yet among the vulgar, from ill-grounded prejudices, and even from religious tenets, it has made very little progress; notwithstanding the earnest admonitions, and gratuitous assistance of medical practitioners."[209]

Opposition to inoculation on religious grounds never entirely died out, and even when the new vaccination was introduced at the beginning of the nineteenth century, there were minor problems on this account; for example, Thomas Warren, curate to the parish of Flamstead and Kensworth in Hertfordshire, wrote as late as 1803 that there were "some people . . . who object to Inoculation altogether, thinking it sinful and presumptious willingly to incur a disease."[210]

Much of the religious opposition that remained however appears to have been linked to attitudes of fatalistic resignation, which flourished particularly in large towns. Haygarth came nearest to explaining this link. He noted that in Chester

"the lower class of people have no fear of the casual [natural] smallpox. Many more examples occurred of their wishes and endeavour to catch the infection, than to avoid it."[211]

Haygarth tried to account for this fatalistic attitude of parents towards their children catching smallpox, and wrote:

"This . . . prejudice . . . probably prevails in other towns, especially in those which are so large as perpetually to nourish the distemper, by so quick a succession of infants as constantly to supply fresh subjects for infection . . . [whereas] . . . in small towns and villages, especially placed in remote situations, the young generation grow up to have a consciousness of the danger before they are attacked by the dreadful disease."[212]

The implication of Haygarth's argument is that the endemic nature of smallpox in the large towns engendered an attitude of fatalistic resignation amongst parents as a result of the inevitable and regular, year-by-year returns of epidemics, whereas in the countryside relatively infrequent epidemics produced a much greater consciousness of the devastations of the disease. There is no logical reason why this should be the case, except that countryside epidemics were much more spectacular than those in the large towns, mainly because a much larger proportion of the total population, including adolescents and young adults, were attacked. The important role of the spectacular nature of countryside epidemics in encouraging inoculation is illustrated by the response to a smallpox epidemic in the Chelmsford area. In 1779 a local surgeon described the practice of inoculation in the locality:

"it has been neglected by the common people for the last 7 or 8 years. It seems as much forgot in many parts of the kingdom as though it had never been known, until the natural small-pox comes with its usual train of malignant disorder and awakens them out of their lethargy. The Faculty, then are hurried into inoculation, perhaps, with too much precipitary, and are under the necessity of complying with the impatience of the people without proper preparations . . ."[213]

This impatience for quick inoculation in response to a threatening epidemic sometimes led to a kind of panic, as in Blandford in 1766 when "a perfect rage for inoculation seized the whole town."[214] The same type of experience was repeated in Hertfordshire in 1770 when an epidemic threatened, for according to Dimsdale, "the poor in my neighbourhood flocked in numbers, beseeching me to" inoculate them.[215]

Although the poor in large towns did not enthusiastically embrace inoculation as they did in the countryside (at least during periods of threatening epidemics), it would be misleading to assume that the town poor were indifferent to the fate of their children as the result of religious or fatalistic resignation. Haygarth himself described a mother in Chester who refused to have her child inoculated, on the grounds that "four of my children have already died of the common [natural] smallpox, and if my remaining child should die by inoculation, I could never forgive myself."[216] This does not indicate a fatalistic resignation so much (and certainly not an "endeavour to catch the infection"), but more a psychological unfamiliarity with the protection given by inoculation. John Franks wrote in 1800 of the London poor:

"when smallpox is in a house where there are many children and adults liable to the disease, the proposal to inoculate gratuitously, all those who are not exempt, is too often disregarded by themselves or relations. It is in vain that we expostulate in these situations, and endeavours to convince them of the non-existence of a double infection [that inoculated children would later catch smallpox], or of an accumulation of disease; for the contrary opinion is too firmly impressed to be easily obliterated."[217]

The problem was to familiarize the urban poor with the benefits of inoculation, and although we shall see later this was more-or-less achieved at the end of the eighteenth and the beginning of the nineteenth centuries, it had occurred much more quickly and effectively in the countryside. The benefits of inoculation were spectacularly obvious in the small towns and villages where everybody could follow the exact course of an epidemic and gain a very personal knowledge of the protective power of inoculation. A writer to *The Monthly Ledger* explained in 1775 the difference between the countryside and large towns in a discussion on inoculation:

"But those who know most of the country know that it is a place where things cannot be secreted, a transaction at ten miles distance is more talked of than a transaction at two streets distance in London."[218]

The medical profession began to make strenuous efforts to spread inoculation in the large towns only towards the end of the eighteenth century. Although the London Smallpox Hospital was founded in 1746 to provide a certain number of charitable inoculations, most other large towns made no charitable provision until as late as the 1780s. It should be remembered that the vast majority of the population lived outside of the large towns during the eighteenth century, and the gradual spread of inoculation in these places will be discussed in the next chapter. As we have seen, the medical profession itself had been originally divided over the subject of inoculation as Mead had noted in 1747,[219] but eight years later, Hosty, who had come to England to study inoculation, reported in 1755:

"Je n'ai pu trouver dans tout Londres un seul Médecin, Chirurgien ou Apoticaire qui s'opposât l'inoculation, ils en sont au contraire tellement partisans qu'ils font tous inoculer leurs propres enfants. Ils regardent cette pratique comme la plus grande découverte que l'on ait en Médecine depuis Hippocrate."[220]

Similarly at about the same time the College of Physicians unanimously approved a formal statement which concluded that inoculation "is at present more generally esteemed and Practised in England than ever, and that they Judge it to be a Practice of the utmost benefit to Mankind."[221]

The remaining factor checking the practice of inoculation was the fear that it would spread smallpox to unprotected people. This invariably led to certain forms of prohibition of the practice (exceptions were made for inoculations in isolated houses), except when an epidemic threatened. Although general inoculation was encouraged when an epidemic threatened, inoculation was frequently discouraged immediately afterwards; the parish of Beaminster near Taunton paid for the inoculation of 379 of its poor in 1791, but immediately afterwards directed that

"from this time Inoculation shall cease in the Town, and if any Surgeon or Apothecary resident in the Town shall set in defiance this Resolution—We shall consider him an improper Person to have Care of the poor at any future Time."[222]

Parish authorities were still frightened that those inoculated would spread the disease to unprotected cases, but they obviously had much less to fear when all the previously unprotected population had been inoculated. This led to what was known as general inoculation, which will be discussed in a separate chapter later. At this point it is sufficient to note that the fear that inoculation would spread smallpox frightened some parish authorities into compelling members of their parish to be inoculated, in order to eliminate the possibility of spreading smallpox. For example, Cowper the poet wrote in 1788:

"the smallpox has done, I believe, all that it has to do at Weston. Old folks, and even women with child, have been inoculated . . . No circumstances whatsoever permitted to exempt the inhabitants of Weston. The old, as well as the young, and the pregnant, as well as they who had themselves within them, have been inoculated . . ."[223]

56

CHAPTER 4

Growth in the Practice of Inoculation

We have seen in the last chapter that inoculation "lost ground" in the 1730s, and before about 1740 was practised only on an insignificant scale. According to the medical historian Moore, writing in 1815, "the American reports [of a more successful form of inoculation] were so encouraging that about the year 1740 the practice was revived by a few surgeons in Portsmouth, Chichester, Guildford, Petersfield and Winchester, and gradually extended in the Southern Counties."[224] The American reports that Moore referred to where the large number of inoculations carried out by Mowbray and Kilpatrick during the 1738 epidemic in Charleston. According to Kilpatrick 800 people were inoculated, of whom eight died, a fatality rate of one per cent. This lower fatality was probably partly due to the improved technique of inoculation associated with the names of Sloane and Ranby; Kilpatrick later claimed in 1754 that an essay of his written in 1743 on the improved technique of inoculation "had been of some effectual tendency to revive the practice."[225] It has recently been argued by one medical historian that Kilpatrick was prone to self-advertisement, leading him to exaggerate his role in the revival of inoculation in England.[226] It is clear, however, that he contributed to the spread of inoculation through publicising its relative success in Charleston.

Inoculation during this period was almost entirely restricted to the rich; the inoculation of the poor near Guildford during the 1740s paid for by "a noble person" was an exception, although it contained the seeds of popular inoculation for the poor:

"Country people came every market day to have the operation performed, then went home, kept themselves warm, drank whine whey, and in eight days took the distemper; and so much success atended the practice, that it was answer to their acquaintance, of 3 or 4 hurrying along the town together, that they were going to be **oculated**."[227]

The inoculation of the poor and the general population became increasingly widespread during the 1750s. We have already noted the surgeon from Chelmsford who wrote in 1753 that "the lower class of people [are] coming into it [inoculation] very fast in these parts."[228] Similarly, Kilpatrick described the beginning of popular inoculation in his book published in 1754, although as a respectable member of the medical profession he was somewhat appalled by this development:

"But since we have certain Accounts that the Populace, who were at first strongly prepossessed against this Practice, and who so rarely stop at the Golden Mean, are rushing into the contrary Extreme, and go promiscuously from different Distances to little Market Towns, where, without any medical Advice, and very little Consideration, they procure Inoculation from some Operator, too often as crude and thoughtless as themselves; congratulating each other after it over strong Liquor, and returning immediately to their ordinary Labour and Way of living . . ."[229]

The operators that Kilpatrick referred to were probably country surgeons and apothecaries, for he discusses them in very critical terms with reference to their role in inoculation; some of these "operators" may also have been amateurs.

Although Kilpatrick accused the populace of "rushing into the contrary Extreme", he himself probably greatly exaggerated the practice of popular inoculation during this period. As late as 1751 the *Gentleman's Magazine* could refer to inoculation as "this new fashionable operation",[230] and it has already been noted how another gentleman observed in 1752 that the "poor in general are absolutely cut off from all share in it . . . and not only the very poor people, but multitudes of others, many farmers and tradesmen . . ."[231] It is partly possible to assess the extent of inoculation by analyzing the overseers-of-the-poor's accounts and contemporary descriptions of particular local inoculations. During a smallpox epidemic at Bradford-on-Avon, Wiltshire in 1752/53, 1,456 people caught natural smallpox while another 127 were inoculated—a small proportion of the total population at risk.[232] Similarly, during an epidemic at Salisbury in 1753, there were 1,309 cases of natural smallpox and 422 inoculated cases, a somewhat larger minority.[233] At Blandford, Dorset, in 1753 there were 309 people inoculated, while only 40 actually died from smallpox; it is not known how many people were at risk of catching the disease (and therefore needed the protection of inoculation), although at the beginning of a similar epidemic 13 years later (in 1766) it was estimated that 700 persons in the town were at risk. As 44 people died from smallpox during the 1766 epidemic and 384 were inoculated, it is reasonable to assume that under 700 people were at risk in 1753, and therefore about a half of the vulnerable population were inoculated in that year.[234] This was a significant proportion and perhaps another example of the same kind is to be found at Wootton-under-Edge, Gloucs., in 1756 when 336 "paupers" were inoculated,[235] although we do not have sufficient information to estimate the proportion of the population at risk who were protected in this way.

The analysis of overseers-of-the-poor's accounts is somewhat misleading in arriving at conclusions about the extent of inoculation during the 1750s, as many parishes did not pay for the inoculation of their poor until well after this period: for example, in Rye, Sussex "this system [of mass inoculation paid for by the parish] was first introduced in 1767", when 329 poor persons were inoculated.[236] We have seen earlier that as late as 1776, Dimsdale stated that some parishes in Hertfordshire refused to pay for the inoculation of those in the parish who could not afford to pay for it themselves. Although Kilpatrick probably exaggerated the extent of the practice of inoculation in the 1750s, there was undoubtedly a change in the attitude of the general population towards inoculation from before 1749 when it

"gained but little credit among the common sort of people, who began to dispute about the lawfulness of propagating diseases, and whether or not the smallpox produced by inoculation would be a certain security against taking it by infection."[237]

to the early 1750s, when they rushed "into the contrary Extreme".

I have previously indicated that inoculation did not become really popular until after the Suttons introduced their improved method of inoculation in the 1760s. This conclusion is confirmed by a statistical estimate of the number of people inoculated in England up until 1766, which according to the medical historian Klebs was 200,000 persons.[238] However this estimate was arrived at, it is unlikely to be very accurate, as some inoculation was performed by amateurs and others who must have been very difficult to include in any systematic survey. Evidence of a more reliable kind is provided in Andrew's monograph on inoculation published in 1765:

"Tho' Inoculation has been introduced into Exeter, and the County of Devon, more than twenty three Years . . . it is still sparingly practised . . . In this City [Exeter], according to the best Calculations I can make, since the Year 1741 there have been about 700 Persons inoculated . . ."[239]

Similarly, a correspondent wrote in the *Monthly Ledger* in 1765:

"I have been witness to the progress of inoculation, from the introduction of the Suttonian method, thro' a very considerable part of a populous country [Hertfordshire]: at the introduction of that method, the subjects obnoxious to the disease [*i.e.* at risk and not protected by inoculation] were more numerous in proportion to the example, than they could possibly be in London at any period."[240]

This correspondent was discussing whether inoculation spread smallpox or not, and used the favourable experience of inoculation in Hertfordshire during 1766-67 as evidence that a similar form of popular inoculation could be used safely in London. The important point here, however, is that inoculation only really became popular in Hertfordshire with the introduction of the Suttonian method. This was discussed by our correspondent as a part of his general argument:

". . . could the prejudiced surmount their prejudices, and the poor surmount their poverty, and inoculation become as general, throughout London, as it was in Hertfordshire, in 1766 and 1767, the article of smallpox, in the first succeeding year's bill of mortality, would, instead of increasing, sink to 100, and, in a year or two more, to less than twenty."[241]

Contemporaries were unanimous that the Suttons had introduced a method of inoculation which quickly became extremely popular. Woodville in his *History of Inoculation* published in 1796, described the impact of the new method as follows:

"A new era in the history of inoculation had now taken place, by the introduction of the Suttonian practice, which in the year 1765 had extended so rapidly in the counties of Essex and Kent as to much interest the public, who were not less surprised by the novel manner in which it was conducted, than by the uninterrupted success with which it was attended upon a prodigious number of persons."[242]

The success of the Suttonian method enhanced the reputation of inoculation in general and accelerated its practice; this is illustrated by the response to the epidemic in Blandford, Dorset in 1766, when "the general success of Inoculation, in other places, had so prejudiced the minds of the people in its favour, that they were perfectly careless and secure about the consequences."[243] This new popularity of variolation spread to all parts of the country, both south and north, as is illustrated by the example of the surrounding countryside of Leeds in 1768, reported in the "Country News" of a Leeds newspaper:

"Inoculation is now in such universal repute that it is thought there are not less than 10,000 people under the care of practitioners in this part of the world. Many farmers and their families have undergone the operation, and there is scarcely an instance of its failing."[244]

This popularity of inoculation was not confined to the wealthy and the middle-class, but also extended to the labouring part of the population. This was reflected in the (somewhat amusing) complaint of the author of a pamphlet on *The Dearness of Corn and Provisions* published in 1767:

"Inoculation for the small-pox has so very much prevailed in the country, that thousands and ten thousands have escaped the fatal effects of that distemper in the natural way: but what are the consequences of so good an invention? No sooner are the lower sort recovered, but they aim (the women especially) to get a servitude in London, or to use their own words **to better themselves;** this is the only objection that can be made to inoculation, and indeed it is one, for before they did not dare to quit the place of their birth for fear of that distemper, so remained honest and useful in the country . . ."[245]

Smallpox was endemic in a place like London, a fact which no doubt did stop people from the country migrating there if they had not previously had smallpox or been inoculated; the important point here, however, is that "the lower sort" were being inoculated in large numbers at about this time. Even as far afield as the Shetland Islands, the Suttonian innovation significantly transformed the practice of inoculation. In 1761 only ten to twelve people had been inoculated, but during the next smallpox epidemic of 1769/1770, a local surgeon "inoculated several hundred, chiefly of the lower class,"[246] after which date inoculation was "performed by a great number of native doctors",[247] including the locally renowned John Williamson.

In order to convey the dramatic nature of the transformation brought about by the Suttons, I will quote at length from a series of letters written by a Mr Thomas Davies, who was bailiff to the Glynde estate in Sussex, to his employer's agent residing in London. These letters give a vivid sense of the popular interest and excitement created by the new mass practice of inoculation, and show that the Suttons had many rivals by the year 1767 (when the letters were written), and that these rivals were often cheaper and sometimes even more effective as inoculators. The following were all written from Glynde, a very small village, at a time when smallpox had just begun to affect neighbouring areas:

"28 Feb. 1767 . . . Even those who have had it [smallpox] themselves, as we expect to be so surrounded with it soon, don't know but they may be a means of bringing home to their families, which is my case. This danger together with the great Success and liberty of moving about and freedom from even Sickness, in the new method, to all Ages and Constitutions, made me wish I could persuade our little Parish to do as Tunbridge Wells and Ryegate and such places have done *i.e.* to inoculate all in order to be clear of it in about a fortnight or three weeks . . . 18 March . . . yesterday an Agreement was made with Mr Watson & Co . . . who have inoculated above 2,000 people this winter about Rye, Winchelsea, Romney and the East of Sussex, with equal Success but less Physicking and more expedition than Sutton or his people. His method is, to innoculate without previous preparation; and physick afterwards as occasion requires . . . The Terms he offered to inoculate us I think is reasonable enough, as he was very desirous of making an Attack on Sutton who innoculated at the Park House and environ, *i.e.* about the Eroyle, little Horstead etc [in the neighbourhood of Glynde]. He undertook as many as would be innoculated of Glynd people for 20 Guineas and if there were not 40 people in all he would not insist on so much . . . I should think it probable we shall have more unless terrified by the Nonsense of our Neighbours. 19 March . . . This day Blackman of Southover came here to hear our Terms, he talked of about 300 in their parish that have not had it and Watson offered to inoculate them all for £100. He supposes they will comply. This will spoil Sutton's Trade in the Pleshut House who takes in none under 6 Guineas and 4 Guineas where the lowest price people are crowded 2 in a Bed and 8 Beds in a room. They clear there at present at the rate of 100 Guineas a Week besides other parties, so that it is high time to pull down their prices; or else they would run away with all the Cash of the Country . . . 14 April . . . There are at least a Score of Inoculating Doctors advertising every week in the Lewes Journal, all in the newest Fashion, and I believe as far as I can hear, all with the same Success. For if but one should happen to die, all the County would soon hear of it. Our Doctor is above advertising and has not once appeared in print. I believe him to be as good as any of them, Sutton & Co not excepted, and I know he is by much more expeditious."[248]

The small parish went on to successfully inoculate its forty or so vulnerable members—the fears of their neighbouring rival parish of Firle that inoculation might spread the natural form of the disease were countered by isolating the inoculated in a special inoculation stable—and one of the many rivals to the Sutton family proved that he was more than their match in inoculating skills (Davies quite correctly realised the advantages of no preparation and minimal "physicking"). We see in Davies's account that the fear that inoculation would spread smallpox was a major incentive for a general inoculation of all vulnerable members of a community—a theme to be discussed in the next chapter—and that this had become a common practice in Sussex by 1767. The Suttons' prices quoted by Davies were the ones charged for private patients undergoing inoculation in one of their special inoculation houses, but as we will now see, the Suttons were forced by the ruthless market forces revealed by

Davies, to significantly lower their prices particularly to the parish poor.

Although Robert Sutton had perfected a much safer technique of inoculation at the beginning of 1762, it was his son Daniel who was responsible for its popularisation. Not only did he inoculated 417 of the "poor" of Maldon, Essex in one day, as well as 70 of the "tradespeople and gentry", to clear the town of smallpox in 1764, but also

> "Several other large parties in Kent, and in various parts of the kingdom have been inoculated in the same manner (as at Maldon), and with the same success."[249]

The numbers inoculated by Daniel Sutton accelerated rapidly during this period; he inoculated 1,629 in 1764, 4,347 in 1765, and 7,613 in 1766. In addition, about 6,000 inoculations were carried out by his assistants who had been "taught . . . his method".[250] Sutton's own number of inoculations were taken from his record books, but the scale of his activity is confirmed by independent evidence from other sources. We have already seen the spectacular success of his mass inoculation at Ewell in Surrey in 1766, and similar feats were performed at Maldon in Essex and elsewhere. Sutton quoted the following example in his book written in 1796:

> "About ten or fifteen years after I had introduced and established the new method of inoculation, I was employed to inoculate a large party, of the same town, consisting of above 700 persons. About one half of them were inoculated before twelve o'clock, and the other half were begun upon, at half past three in the afternoon: They were all inoculated by my own hand, from the same individual subject . . . the medicines were procured from the same druggist . . ."[251]

I have already suggested that these mass inoculations performed in one day usually took place amongst the ordinary population, with wealthier parishioners insisting on the more expensive and medically orthodox period of preparation etc. Although Sutton performed all the inoculations himself in the example quoted above, it is clear that he employed assistants to do much of the work for him; according to Woodville, Sutton's "practice in Kent [before 1767] being also very extensive, he was under the necessity of employing several medical assistants."[252] By 1796, Sutton could claim to have been involved in "of near 100,000 instances of inoculation, in which I have been either immediately employed, or have had some concern, in consultation with others."[253] There is, however, some ambiguity about who these other inoculators were. I have previously mentioned that the Sutton family set up a series of partnerships in all parts of the country. Houlton described in 1768 how this came about:

"Every paper throughout the kingdom echoed with its [the Suttonian method's] success. Eminent physicians and surgeons were daily applying to the family to be appointed partners for particular counties, or for foreign parts. Connections have been made with many gentlemen of the faculty, while others continue still to apply for that purpose."[254]

He then listed all members of the Sutton family (six sons and two sons-in-law of Robert Sutton) and partners who were "authorised" members of the enterprise at the time of publication in 1768:[255]

Mr Robert Sutton, sen.	Framingham Earl, Norfolk
Mr Robert Sutton, jun. Joseph Power, M.D. partner	} Paris
Messrs Dan. Sutton / Will. Sutton / Peale, partner	} London
Mr Joseph Sutton / Gamble, partner	} Oxford
Mr Tho. Sutton	Newport, Isle of Wight
Mr Jas. Sutton	Wakefield, Yorkshire
Mr Hewitt, son-in-law to Mr Sutton / Alex Sutherland, M.D. partner	} Hague
Mr Shuttleworth, son-in-law	Birmingham
Messrs Robard / Ford / Ludlow	} Bristol
Mr Read	Gloucester
Mr Vaux	Hereford
Mr Vaux, junior	Worcester
Messrs Tatum / Wick	} Salisbury } Wiltshire
Mr Jones / Mr Marsh	Bradford / Highworth
Messrs Smiths / Mr Jones	Winchester / Portsmouth } Hampshire
Messrs Sampson / Jay	Sherborne / Maiden Newton } Dorset
Mr Assey	Taunton, Somerset

Messrs Bromley	Exeter	} Devon
Hooper	Plymouth	
Mr Campble	Truro, Cornwall	
Mr Steed	Ingatestone, Essex	
Mr Buck	Ipswich, Suffolk	
Mr Argles	Wisbech, Cambridgeshire	
Messrs Byre	Chertsey	
Newland	Guildford	} Surrey
Kerr	Dorking	
Mr Barnwell		Sussex
Messrs Levet	} Buckingham	
Saunders		
Dent	}	Buckingham-
Terriers		shire
Mr Bond		Northampton-
		shire
Mr Richardson		Huntingdon-
		shire
Messrs Bevil	Manchester	} Lancashire
Goodwin	Liverpool	
Mr Lynn	Shrewsbury, Shropshire	
John Denman, M.D.	Bakewell, Derbyshire	
Tho. Rutherford, M.D.		Durham
Messrs Lyde	Brecknockshire	} Wales
Bevan	Glamorganshire	
Messrs Houlton	} Dublin	} Ireland
Blake		
Sparrow		
John Harley, M.D.	Cork	
John Morgan, M.D.	Strabane, Tyrone	
Messrs Vachell	Soon to be appointed	
Ward	to particular districts	
Shields	In Ireland	
Arnold		
Mr Jewitt	Jamaica	
Mr Smith	Virginia	

The Suttons and their partners were to be found in most counties of England at this time. This laid the foundation for the almost universal practice of the Suttonian method of inoculation in England, so that a correspondent to the *Gentleman's Magazine* in 1796 could write:

"It is now 30 years since the Suttons and others under their instruction, had practised the art of inoculation upon half the kingdom . . ."[256]

It was for this reason that inoculation was referred to as the Suttonian system during a Parliamentary debate in 1808. In 1806 Lipscomb claimed that "Mr Dan. Sutton and his brothers . . . are still living to prove that they have inoculated more than five hundred thousand persons with uniform success."[257] It is impossible to be sure whether this claimed number of inoculations included those performed by partners as well as actual members of the Sutton family, although this is unlikely given the spread of even more popular forms of inoculation which would have made partnership with the Suttons (and therefore the use of their name) increasingly irrelevant. The relative decline in the fortunes of the Sutton family can be traced in the history of Daniel's practice. According to Woodville,

"In 1767, Mr D. Sutton removed to London, where he hoped to profit by his profession still more than he had done in the country; but his practice fell far short of his expectations; and the two houses, one at Kensington Gore, and another at Brentford, which were procured for his inoculated patients, were soon abandoned."[258]

This suggests that Sutton failed as an inoculator in London, and his eclipse from the fame he acquired during the 1760s is reflected in a pathetic advertisement that he put in the front of his book in 1796:

"I find it has been circulated, That I am not the person who introduced the New System of Inoculation . . . that for many years I had quitted my profession, and was long since dead."[259]

The main reason for this decline I have discussed previously, i.e. Sutton's unwillingness to abandon preparation and associated medical treatment, and the relatively high cost of his practice. He was displaced by more popular inoculators who simplified the method of inoculation to its logical conclusion, and reduced its price. However there was another reason why he did not succeed in establishing a fashionable practice in London:

"The terms of Sutton are so moderate that men in mean circumstances, men of low education and dissolute life, repair to his house, which is so confused and disorderly a place that one would admire one-tenth part of his patients do not perish by their irregularities."[260]

We do not have to take this elegant disdain too literally to recognize that Sutton was no longer attracting the wealthier type of client. The Suttons had obviously made a great deal of money out of inoculation—Daniel Sutton is reputed to have made 6,000 guineas between 1763 and 1766[261]—and they appear to have sold the "secret" of their method to their partners for between fifty and one hundred pounds, or a half share in the profits.[262] He seems to have missed his chance of lasting fame and wealth when he refused to go to Russia to inoculate Empress Catherine II— Dimsdale, who successfully performed the operation, was made a Baron of the Russian Empire, awarded a sum of £10,000 and an annuity of £500.[263] The reasons for Sutton's refusal are unknown; he may have been frightened of the consequences of failure with someone of such eminent status. It is clear he very soon concentrated on the inoculation of the ordinary population as was reflected in the following advertisement:

> "Sutton-House, London, Jan. 20, 1770. The many thousands of industrious poor, who have past happily through the Small-Pox by Inoculation, under the direction of Mr Daniel Sutton . . . induce him to offer to the public, the following more extensive plan . . . Convenient houses, in different parts of the Town (each being inhabited by a reputable Surgeon or Apothecary, instructed by him) are engaged—that to these houses he proposes such patients as have tickets of recommendation from subscribers, are to repair on the day and hour appointed in the said tickets, in order to receive preparatory medicines and instructions, they will be informed, when to return to be inoculated . . when they will finally receive such medicines and ample directions for their conduct, during the progress of their disease, at their own habitations, as will render any further attendance unnecessary . . . This plan is principally intended for the benefit of the industrious poor; such as the families of artificers, handicraftsmen, servants, labourers, etc."[264]

It is not known how successful this plan was, although clearly it must have had only limited success for Sutton's virtual eclipse by 1796 (although he was still practising by then). However, we cannot assume that the plan was a total failure, for according to Gorton's Biographical Dictionary, "Daniel simplified and improved his father's mode of practice, and settled first at Ingatestone, Essex, and afterwards in London, where he was very successful."[265] If we take Sutton's own claims to the numbers inoculated by him and his assistants, it is possible to trace the change in extent of his practice. Between 1763 and 1766 he claimed to have inoculated about 20,000 people and by 1796 a total of 100,000; during the first period he was inoculating about 6,700 people a year, whereas between 1766 and 1796 the average number was about 2,700. It is unlikely that his London plan could have succeeded on any extensive scale, owing to the expense and inconvenience involved for the poor, as well as the necessity of being recommended by a subscriber; in this respect the plan was similar to that of the London Smallpox Hospital, which was only a limited success for the same reasons. Sutton, of course, did not confine his activities to London as was demonstrated by his inoculation of "a large party, of the same town, consisting of above 700 persons" at some time during the late 1770s. Whatever the fate of Daniel Sutton's individual practice, it is clear that the Sutton family as a whole, along with their partners, continued to practice inoculation on an extensive scale until at least the end of the eighteenth century. There is evidence for this conclusion independent of the Sutton family itself; for example, Fewster, a surgeon in Thornbury, Gloucs., wrote in 1798:

"The late Mr Grove was a very extensive Smallpox inoculator, frequently having 200 to 300 patients at one time . . . Mr Grove and myself formed a connection with Mr Sutton, the celebrated inoculator . . ."[266]

It is not clear whether this type of partner was included by the Suttons when they made claims of the numbers inoculated by them, the wording of their statements often being ambiguous. For example, Robert Sutton claimed in an advertisement published in 1777 "that in the SUTTONIAN PRACTICE, which has been established nearly thirty years . . . nearly three hundred thousand persons have happily passed through smallpox [i.e. been inoculated] . . ."[267]

In 1763, Houlton stated that the Suttons had inoculated about fifty-five thousand people (with only six deaths),[268] and we have previously seen that it was claimed in 1806 that "Dan. Sutton and his brothers . . . have inoculated more than five hundred thousand persons." If these statistics were reliable and referred to the same type of practitioner (i.e. either just the Suttons or the Sutton family plus partners throughout), they would indicate a decline in the extent of the practice after 1777. The average number of yearly inoculations according to these figures was about 27,200 between 1768 and 1777, and approximately 6,900 between 1777 and 1806. It is unlikely however that these statistics do refer to all the inoculations performed under the "Suttonian system", as it must have been almost impossible for the Suttons to collect returns of numbers inoculated by all their partners. This point is illustrated by the fact that Fewster, the surgeon referred to above, who was a partner of the Suttons, was very vague about the number of inoculations that he carried out; if he had kept statistical records he no doubt would have quoted them in connection with the point that he was making. No statistics can ultimately measure the importance of the Suttons, as their method greatly influenced practitioners such as Dimsdale, and less well-known local surgeons, apothecaries and amateur inoculators who spread the method, until finally inoculation itself was referred to as the Suttonian system.

Howlett summed up the general position in 1781 with reference to the extent of inoculation:

"In provincial towns and villages, as soon as this disorder [smallpox] makes its appearance, inoculation takes place amongst all ranks of people; the rich and poor, from either choice or necessity, almost instantly have recourse to it."[269]

Howlett's reference to "from either choice or necessity" probably referred to the existence of compulsory inoculation in some parishes. I have already noted Cowper's description of compulsory inoculation at Weston, Norfolk in 1788; apparently it was possible for the parish authorities to exercise compulsory powers through their control of poor relief, although obviously this type of compulsion would not apply to richer parishioners.[270] It is impossible to give an exact account of the extent of inoculation by this period, as there are no reliable, comprehensive statistics available; however, it is clear from all the evidence cited (including examples of general and mass inoculations mentioned in previous chapters and to be discussed in the next chapter) that inoculation was practised very extensively in the countryside by about 1780. That this was not only a function on the reduction of cost is illustrated by the history of inoculation in Beaminster, Dorset. In 1758 at a Vestry meeting,

"It was agreed and Ordered that Mr Oliver Hoskins, Mr Jms. Daniel and Mr Jms. Cox shall be paid and Allow'd for Inoculating, Attending and Supplying Physick to all such Poor Parishioners as are willing to be Inoculated after the Rate of Five shillings p. head . . ."[271]

The result was that £6.15.0d was "paid for Inoculating 27 poor at 5/- each." This sum must be contrasted with that paid out in 1780 to John Daniel, John Cox and James David who each received "£17.13.4d for Inoculating the Poor." Similarly in 1791 a total of £66.6.6d was paid for the inoculation of 379 poor people, at three shillings and sixpence per head.[272] The population of Beaminster was 1,708 in 1775 according to a local census, and assuming a birth rate of 35 per 1,000, about 60 children were born into the parish every year. Between 1780 and 1791 there would have been about 660 children born into the parish, some of which would have died from diseases other than smallpox between the two dates. The inoculation of 379 poor persons in 1791, suggests that the majority of the population at risk, (mostly children in this case) were inoculated and thus protected against attacks of natural smallpox by the end of the eighteenth century; from all the evidence taken together it is justifiable to conclude that inoculation protected the majority of the population at risk from at least as early as 1780 in Beaminster.

Ironically, one of the best pieces of general evidence for the extent of the practice of inoculation in the country at large came from the pen of Edward Jenner. In his *Inquiry* written in 1798, he stated that the prophylactic powers of cowpox had probably first been noticed with "the general introduction of inoculation,"[273] and elaborated on this in his pamphlet on the origin of vaccine inoculation published in 1801:

"My inquiry into the nature of Cow Pox commenced upwards of twenty-five years ago. My attention to this singular disease was first excited by observing, that among those whom in the country I was frequently called upon to inoculate, many resisted every effort to give them the Small Pox. These patients I found had undergone a disease they called the Cow Pox . . . a vague opinion prevailed that it was a preventive of the Small Pox. This opinion I found was, comparatively, new among them; for all the older farmers declared that they had no such idea in their early days—a circumstance that seemed easily to be accounted for, from my knowing that the common people were very rarely inoculated for the Small Pox, till that practice was rendered general by the improved method introduced by the Suttons. So that the working people in the dairies were seldom put to the test of the preventive powers of the Cow Pox."[274]

In fact, Jenner's claims for his new type of inoculation were very modest in his first publication on the subject. He saw it merely as an improvement on an existing practice which was highly successful and very widespread:

"Should it be asked whether this investigation is a matter of mere curiosity, or whether it tends to any beneficial purpose? I should answer, that notwithstanding the happy effects of Inoculation, with all the improvements which the practice has received since its first introduction into this country, it not very unfrequently produces deformity of the skin, and sometimes, under the best management, proves fatal."[275]

Jenner himself had of course been a variolator for many years, and was in a position from personal experience to reach the above conclusion about the history of inoculation in the second half of the eighteenth century (he had been inoculated as a boy in 1756).

Nearly all contemporaries were unanimous that inoculation was very extensively practised in the countryside but greatly neglected in the large towns; for example, Watkinson wrote in 1777 that "since the year 1755 . . . inoculation, tho' much practised in the country parts of England, made no progress in the capital."[276] The neglect of inoculation in London is confirmed by Black who wrote in 1781 that "inoculation at the expiration of sixty years, since its first introduction, has made very little progress in London."[277] We have seen previously that the neglect of inoculation was also prevalent in other large towns during this period. In 1774 Aikin described the severe smallpox epidemic in Warrington which had taken place in the previous year; he noted:

> "Not ten, I believe, were inoculated in the whole town and neighbourhood: these all did well, yet their example was not sufficient to overcome some accidental prejudices taken against it."[278]

Similarly Percival noted in 1773 that "inoculation is not much practised here" in Manchester.[279] The initial reaction of medical observers to the slow spread of inoculation in the large towns (as against its rapid spread in the countryside) is illustrated by the following statement made by Haygarth in 1780:

> "And it cannot be supposed that the inhabitants of towns are more ignorant or more obstinate [than those living in the countryside]. There is not a reasonable doubt that our poor fellow-citizens would eagerly and universally embrace a proposal to preserve [by inoculation] their children from death and deformity, if the intelligent and opulent would humanely exert their influence and assistance to carry it into execution."[280]

Haygarth was referring to the fact that there was little or no free provision of inoculation in the large towns.

The only large town with an institution providing charitable inoculation was London—the London Smallpox Hospital was founded in 1746 partly to provide inoculation for the poor. However, as no person under the age of seven was inoculated by the hospital, the vast majority of the population at risk (in London practically all cases of smallpox occurred amongst children under the age of seven) was excluded automatically. For a poor person to be inoculated at the hospital, it was necessary for him to be recommended by one of the subscribers to the charity. It appears that the hospital was partly founded and used during the earlier period by the wealthy of London for the inoculation of their servants, many of whom were migrants from the countryside.[281] There is no evidence that any of the parish authorities in the large towns made provision for the inoculation of their poor as was the universal practice in the countryside. This raises an interesting question as to why there was this difference between large town and countryside (possibly due to the much larger numbers that the town parish authorities had to deal with?), which is beyond the scope of this book. The first person to attempt to remedy this situation in the towns was Lettsom, who established a London society for inoculating the poor in their own homes in 1775. He described the background to the events leading up to the establishment of the society and its effects as follows:

". . . to a very useful, and the most numerous part of the [London] community, the advantages resulting from it [inoculation] have hitherto in great measure been lost, either from the confined circumstances of the poor, or from their prejudices against so extraordinary an innovation in practice. At length, however, examples of the dreadful effects of the natural, and the wonderful success of the artificial disease [inoculation], have overcome these ill-founded prejudices, and nothing seemed wanting, to enable the poor to reap the benefit of this practice, but an establishment suited to their condition and circumstances . . . no institution for that purpose existed here till the year 1775, when the Society for General Inoculation of the Poor was first established . . . The poor, however, though slow in admitting new improvements, are not soon to be reasoned out of self-evident facts, and their willingness to try Inoculation continues to augment with the success of the practice."[262]

It appears that Lettsom's plan of general inoculation of the poor in London was having considerable success, but it was unfortunately thwarted by the opposition of Dimsdale who argued that the inoculation of children in their own homes would spread smallpox through the over-populated courts and alley-ways. Lettsom, instead of retorting that "most born in London have the smallpox before they are seven" anyway (a fact confirmed by subsequent statistical study), engaged Dimsdale in a bitter polemical dispute. As we have seen, Lettsom's main argument was that no "instance occurred to the medical practitioners engaged in this institution, to prove that the infection has been propagated from an inoculated patient."[283] It was unnecessary as an argument, for even if inoculation spread smallpox it would have been irrelevant in a situation like London where the disease was already endemic. Lettsom attempted to organise popular inoculation for the poor in London a second time in 1779, but this too failed, mainly through Dimsdale's opposition.[284] The only provision of free inoculation for the poor in London until the beginning of vaccination was that provided by the London Smallpox Hospital.[285] It did increase significantly its number of inoculations (particularly after the adoption of the Suttonian method), partly through allowing the inoculation of out-patients and lowering the minimum age to five years. According to an account of the hospital's history written in 1830, there were

48,062 people inoculated by the hospital between 1746 and 1822 when the practice was discontinued.[286] This is an average of about 632 inoculations per year throughout the whole period, which of course is insignificant in a town like London with a population of something like 800,000 (assuming a birth-rate of 35 per 1,000, about 28,000 children would be born every year). It is difficult to know how popular inoculation became in London through the practice of Daniel Sutton and other private inoculators, as there is so little evidence available. Watkinson stated in 1777 that "inoculation has become very fashionable" in London during "the last four years".[287] The fashion must have largely excluded the London poor, for as we saw in the last chapter, Franks found great prejudice amongst them against inoculation as late as 1800. Evidence arising out of the polemical dispute between the supporters of the new vaccination and the old inoculation at the beginning of the nineteenth century, indicates that there was a fairly marked change in popular attitude at the turn of the century. According to a report in the *Gentleman's Magazine* in 1803:

"Mr. Wilberforce observed on the popular prejudice, that, out of 100 who had been vaccinated at the Smallpox Hospital, not five would have submitted, had they not supposed it to have been the old-fashioned mode of Inoculation."[288]

Similarly Jenner wrote to Lettsom in 1807 about an interview with Mr. Percival

"with the sole view of inquiring whether it was the intention of Government to give a check to the licentious manner in which small-pox inoculation at this time was conducted in the Metropolis."[289]

Adams confirmed this upsurge of inoculation, and wrote that it "increased to such a degree [in London], as to alarm many well intentioned people."[290] This and similar evidence makes it quite clear that inoculation was very extensively practised in London by the beginning of the nineteenth century, and this practice extended to the ordinary population. The popular support of inoculation in London was associated with an opposition to vaccination and when Jenner was awarded £20,000 by Parliament for his discovery of vaccination, John Gale Jones the radical leader and an apothecary, sent a message to Jenner at his lodgings in Bedford Place to advise him "immediately to quit London, for there was no knowing what an enraged populace might do."[291] Jenner had urged the Government to suppress inoculation, and occasional convictions of inoculators for "spreading smallpox" did occur; for example, according to one report in 1815:

"Another conviction has taken place of a person, of the name of Burnett, practising as an Apothecary etc. in London, (who held out the lure of gratuitous inoculation), for ordering children to be exposed in the streets while under smallpox, whereby the infection was disseminated. He was sentenced, to six months imprisonment."[292]

There is no need to stress the unfairness of this conviction, for it must have been scientifically impossible to discover whether Burnett's inoculations did spread smallpox or not in a place like London where natural smallpox was endemic. The important point here is that inoculation was very extensively practised amongst the ordinary population of London by the beginning of the nineteenth century.

Inoculation became popular in other large towns at an earlier date than it did in London, and this was mainly due to the establishment of special institutions for the inoculation of the poor. Haygarth summarized the position in 1793 when he discussed methods of eliminating smallpox:

"That, in large towns, inoculation, at stated periods must be performed, as already practised in Chester, Liverpool, Newcastle, Leeds, Dumfries etc."[293]

Free general inoculations first occurred in Leeds and Liverpool in 1781. There was a severe smallpox epidemic in Leeds, and during the first six months of 1781, 462 young children were attacked and 130 died; the plan of general inoculation was then adopted and during the next six months 385 were inoculated. Although this number of inoculations appears minute in a town like Leeds with a population of 17,117, it is important to understand that smallpox was virtually endemic in such towns and therefore the population at risk was only a fraction of the total population, *i.e.* infants and very young children who were born after the previous epidemic (epidemics occurred every year in these towns). It was found by survey that there were only 700 persons (children) who had not been previously infected with smallpox in Leeds by the middle of 1781; 385 of these 700 were inoculated during the latter half of the year.[294] Very little else is known about inoculation in Leeds, except that there was at least a second attempt at some kind of general inoculation in 1788. Lucas, one of the surgeons to the General Infirmary at Leeds, discussed this inoculation in an account published in the *Gentleman's Magazine* in 1790:

"I had no sooner taken down the names of such children as offered for inoculation [March 1788], than I was requested by several persons to extend the same privilege throughout the parish. As such a plan exceeded my intended limits, I acquainted a noble Lord with my proceedings, who immediately approved what had been done, and, in the most polite manner, requested that he might be at the sole expence of executing a scheme which every family to whom he had applied had, not many years before, peremptorily refused. Notwithstanding a few private patients, near eighty were inoculated, without even any apparent danger; whilst two out of five who caught the natural infection died."[295]

This illustrates the unsatisfactory nature of the type of provision of inoculation in some of the large towns. Unlike small towns and villages, only sporadic attempts were made at general inoculation, and these sometimes only when there was financial backing from a charitably disposed local inhabitant of wealth. Clearly such infrequent "general" inoculations were inadequate in a large town like Leeds, which really required them every year. However, the success of these "general" inoculations (in terms of the immediate saving of life) is likely to have led to the adoption of private inoculation of the poor through the practice of apothecaries, amateurs and parents (as in Canterbury and East Anglia). The "general" inoculation at Liverpool was less successful, for out of "about three or four thousand liable to the disease" in 1781, only 417 were inoculated gratuitously and 100 more in private practice.[296] There was a second gratuitous inoculation in Liverpool in the following spring of 1782, but nothing is known of further inoculations after that date, except what Curril wrote to Haygarth in 1791:

"I lament much that our [Liverpool's] plan for general inoculation is dormant at present, but I hope it will be revived. Our experience, for several years, was uniformly in favour of its utility."[297]

Curril referred to the practice of general inoculation "for several years", which indicates that the inoculations of 1781 and 1782 were subsequently repeated. Also we must not assume that inoculation ceased to be practised in Liverpool in 1791; it might have been the case that there had not been a recent severe epidemic to provide the necessary incentive to inoculation. I have already quoted such a case in Essex in 1779, and it was stated generally to be the case by a medical observer in 1807:

"Unless, therefore, from the immediate dread of epidemic Small-pox, neither Vaccination nor Inoculation appear at any time to have been general, and when the cause of the terror has passed by, the Public have relapsed into a state of indifference and apathy, and the salutary practice has come to a stand . . ."[298]

The most systematic attempt to inoculate regularly each year in a large town occurred in Newcastle; Dr John Clark, applied Lettsom's ideas of general inoculation in the homes of the poor, and between 1786 and 1801 there were 3,268 children inoculated gratuitously by the Newcastle Dispensary.[299] This is an average of just over 200 inoculations a year, which must have protected only a minority of the population at risk, although this population was confined to young children as was reflected in the ages of those inoculated: of 1,056 inoculated during the four-and-a-half years 1786-1790, only 73 were above the age of five and nearly a half (460) were infants under the age of one.[300] It has been previously noted how in Newcastle (1792) "especially among the lower classes, a great and general prejudice against the practice of inoculation" existed. There is no evidence that this prejudice had greatly diminished by the end of the eighteenth century, although private inoculation by apothecaries and others may have become increasingly popular. There were other dispensaries which steadily offered gratuitous inoculation to the children of the poor: those at Whitehaven, where there were 1,079 inoculations from 1783 to 1796, Bath and Chester.[301] Haygarth was responsible for starting free inoculation of the poor in Chester and between the Spring of 1780 and September 1782 there were 213 poor children inoculated as well as 203 done privately.[302] This is an average of about 200 inoculations a year; of a total population of 14,713 in Chester in 1774, 1,060 had not had smallpox and were therefore in need of protection. Assuming the years 1780-82 to have been similar to 1774, nearly forty per cent of the population at risk were inoculated.[303] Haygarth claimed in 1793 that the poor were generally indifferent to inoculation—although later we will see that he probably exaggerated this:

> "In Chester, the lower class of people have no fear of the casual small-pox. Many more examples occurred of their wishes and endeavour to catch the infection, than to avoid it."[304]

The most successful practice of inoculation in a large town of which a detailed description is available, was that in Carlisle. John Heysham, physician to the Carlisle Dispensary which was founded in 1782, gave a year-by-year account of epidemics and the progress of inoculation between 1779 and 1787 in Carlisle and the surrounding neighbourhood. This account is of sufficient importance, to be quoted at some length:

> "1779 . . . several hundreds were inoculated in the neighbourhood of Carlisle, and it is a pleasing truth, that not one of them died . . . Yet so great is the prejudice against the salutary practice of inoculation amongst the vulgar [in Carlisle], that few, very few, can be prevailed upon, either by promises, rewards, or intreaties, to submit to the operation . . .

1781. Great numbers were inoculated both in town and country villages.

1783. In September and October, the small pox became so general, and were of so fatal a kind, that the monthly committee of the dispensary were of opinion, that a general inoculation of the poor and indigent inhabitants, would be attended with very beneficial effects. Early in the month of November, a general inoculation accordingly took place. Great numbers were inoculated, not only by the surgeon to the dispensary, but also by most of the other surgeons in the town.

1785. Early in the month of December, 1784, the small pox were introduced by some vagrants . . . As soon as the disease made its appearance within the walls of the city, the monthly committee of the dispensary resolved, that a general inoculation of the poor inhabitants, agreeable to the plan which I proposed in the year 1783, should take place at the dispensary, and it was with great pleasure I observed the prejudices of the vulgar against that most salutary invention, were greatly diminished. For as soon as the resolution of the committee was made public by the town crier, great number from all quarters of the town flocked to the dispensary, to reap the benefits which it held out of them . . . So that upon a moderate calculation, the whole number inoculated this year, amounted to two hundred; every one of whom—recovered.

1787. The small-pox made their appearance in January, and were in Carlisle the greatest part of the year; but inoculation soon became general, which prevented the disorder from raging with any great degree of violence . . . Eighty-four were inoculated at the dispensary, all of whom not only survived, but had the disorder very favourably; and considerable numbers were likewise inoculated by several surgeons in the town."[305]

The protection which inoculation gave the population at risk in Carlisle was reflected in a sharp decrease in the numbers dying from smallpox, which will be discussed later. Heysham estimated that 300 children caught smallpox in 1779, and if we take this number to be the approximate population at risk in 1785, when Heysham estimated that a total of 200 had been inoculated, it is clear that a majority (about two-thirds) were protected by inoculation in 1785. It is of some interest to note that according to Heysham in 1779 the population of the villages surrounding Carlisle were already practising inoculation quite generally, while in Carlisle itself the ordinary population was still prejudiced against the practice. This difference between country and town did not disappear at any time during the eighteenth century, even in a town like Carlisle (although two-thirds of the population at risk were inoculated in 1785), and this was reflected in a statement made by the medical writer Walker in 1790:

> "Of late, physicians have made a distinction between **partial** and **general** inoculation. Partial, is the mode in which inoculations are carried on at present in the metropolis, and all the capital towns of Great Britain, where everyone who favours the measure, puts it in practice at his own conveniency. General inoculation supposes an agreement of the whole inhabitants to have their children, and all susceptible of the disease, inoculated in one day, a measure which only can be practised in villages and small towns."[306]

It is possible to learn a great deal about the practice of inoculation at the end of the eighteenth and the beginning of the nineteenth century by studying the spread of vaccination. One thing that has always puzzled medical historians is the fact that vaccination was very much less popular in England than it was on the Continent. This is illustrated by a question asked by the Royal College of Physicians in its inquiry on vaccination published in 1807:

> "Why the Practice of Vaccination has not been more generally adopted, especially less so in this country than abroad?"[307]

The answer to this question is to be found in the evidence submitted to the College. It was noted that vaccination made little headway in those areas (*i.e.* outside the large towns) where inoculation was generally practised; for example,

> "The Reports from the professional members of this Society resident in different parts of the County of Somerset universally represent the almost insuperable Difficulties attending their attempts to diffuse the benefits of vaccination owing to the powerful prejudices of the lower classes of the people and also describe the destructive extent to which the practice of Variolous Inoculation is carried on by several persons, some not of the Medical profession . . ."[308]

We do not have to pay too much attention to the critical language used about inoculation, as such language was common to both the supporters of vaccination and inoculation owing to the polemical nature of the dispute. Vaccination was much more popular in the large towns; from Manchester it was reported that

> "The lower classes also **in large towns**, where they can be vaccinated gratis at the public Charities, avail themselves pretty generally of this advantage."[309]

On the present argument, the reason for this was that inoculation had never been universally popular in these large towns as it had been in the country. There was a very specific reason why those familiar with the benefits of inoculation rejected vaccination. From Leeds it was reported in 1801 that

"a very intelligent Practitioner, about seven or eight Miles from Leeds, to whom I sent [vaccine] Matter, and who has inoculated [vaccinated] 150 children in the new Mode, informs me, that a Child, whom he had, a Year before, inoculated for the Cow Pock, and who went thro' the progressive and regular Stages of that mild Disease, has lately been seized with the natural Smallpox which prevailed epidemically in the Village . . . he has had too much Experience in this Way, that he asserts the fact as clear as decisive . . . The Practice [of vaccination] has, however, from such Rumours, declined considerably, and we are now but little in the habit of it in this place, many giving the preference to the inoculated Small Pox."[310]

Contemporaries familiar with inoculation expected to be protected for a lifetime, and vaccination only protected for relatively short periods, although it significantly mitigated the severity of attacks even in the longer period. This affected not only the general population but also the medical profession itself, most of whom had been initially enthusiastic supporters of vaccination:

"very lately [1807] the Small Pox appeared in several parts of Devonshire and Somersetshire, where Vaccination had been practised, and the people insisted on Inoculation, with which some of the Faculty were obliged to comply, seeing the infection spread so fast. That Mr. Goss, of Dawlish, had resorted to a general inoculation, and had submitted his own children, whom he had formerly vaccinated, to the test, two of whom received the Small Pox, and one resisted it."[311]

Mr. Goss submitted his children to the test by inoculating them, and on two of the three children the inoculation took; contemporaries assumed that this meant that such children were not protected by vaccination against natural smallpox. The limited protection given by vaccination (against future attacks) led to Jenner's reputation deteriorating, even amongst his early wealthy supporters, and he wrote in 1811:

"And now this single, solitary instance [Lord Grosvenor's son caught smallpox 10 years after being vaccinated] has occurred, all my past labours, and the result of those labours are forgotten, and I am held up by many, perhaps the majority of the higher Classes, as an object of derision and Contempt."[312]

Jenner was under-stating the number of such cases, although it might have been the first one amongst the aristocracy. The result of contemporary disappointment with vaccination was the continuation of the practice of variolation. Generally, the medical profession continued to be strongly in favour of vaccination, while the population at large—particularly in country areas—remained attached to the old inoculation. For example,

> "The small-pox was accidently introduced into the village of Luddington in the year 1815. A gentleman who was the overseer of the parish immediately endeavoured, in conjunction with Mr Pritchard [senior surgeon to the Stratford-On-Avon dispensary], to persuade the poor of that village to have their children vaccinated. But with the exception of one family, and of one individual in another family, all the poor inhabitants were obstinately determined to have their children inoculated for small-pox; and, with the exception of one infant, they had them inoculated accordingly."[313]

Other examples were found at Wickforn, Berkshire in 1821, where out of a total of 51 children involved, 48 were inoculated, and only three vaccinated,[314] and Aston Cantlow near Henley in Warwickshire in about 1816, when only one of 75 people chose vaccination in preference to inoculation—and then only because the doctor allowed him to continue drinking ale in the one and not the other. (He later changed his mind and was inoculated.)[315]

The persistence of inoculation in East Anglia was brought out in some detail by Cross in his study of the small-pox epidemic which occurred in Norwich in 1820. In some areas inoculation was "practised entirely by old women and a Druggist", whereas in another region centring on Norfolk "itinerant inoculators, irregular practitioners and old women introduced and extended the disease to all quarters by inoculation."[316] Cross, like most of his medical contemporaries was deeply hostile to inoculation by this time, and was shocked to find that in one Hundred made up of 22 parishes, "12 of these were inoculating gratuitously"—and was even more shocked to discover "that several persons of the lower class, some of the inhabitants of Work-houses, were going about the country inoculating."[317] The dilemma that popular demand for inoculation put the medical profession into, was revealed as follows:

> "Many medical men, desirous of doing their duty by discouraging variolous inoculation, have been placed in the most unpleasant situations, and not unfrequently have been

compelled to commit an act which they believed to be im-
moral and injurious, because they could not afford to sacri-
fice the small emmolument arising from it; some have re-
luctantly inoculated whole parishes of the poor, at the
instigation or order of an overseer."[318]

Vaccination was clearly resisted in many areas because
of the preference for the old inoculation, and in some places the
new operation was not introduced for several years after Jenner's
first announcement of his discovery. Dr Forbes, senior physician
to the Chichester Dispensary and a supporter of vaccination,
gave a very detailed description of the history of inoculation and
vaccination in the Chichester area from 1806 until 1821, which
indicates the general position of prophylactic measures taken
against smallpox during the first two decades of the nineteenth
century:

"The last general inoculation for small-pox that took place
in the city of Chichester and neighbourhood was in 1806;
six years later, a considerable number were inoculated in
Havant and Emsworth, and the vicinity, but since that time,
variolous inoculation has been nearly unknown throughout
the district. A few cases of small-pox have, at different times,
been introduced by strangers, and a few of the Practitioners
in the country have occasionally inoculated a small number
of persons, but the occurrence of these solitary cases has
tended rather to increase the practice of vaccination than
to spread the small-pox: and the general fact, on the break-
ing out of the late epidemic [1821], certainly was—that
nearly all the children born in this district since the period
above mentioned, had either been vaccinated, or left entirely unprotected from the infection of small-pox. Owing
to the prejudices and thoughtlessness of the common people,
vaccination had certainly been much less practised than it
ought to have been; being, in a very considerable degree
confined to the children of the upper and middle classes.
The relative proportion of children vaccinated, and those
left unprotected, during the period that has elapsed since
the abolition of variolous inoculation, may be, in some measure, estimated from the facts—that about 500 have been
annually vaccinated by all Surgeons of the district, before
the present year, and that between 2 and 3,000 were vaccinated, and about an equal number inoculated, during the
panic of the late epidemic."[319]

Nearly a half of those inoculated during 1821 had been previously vaccinated (this was the result of distrust of the power of
vaccination to protect against future attacks of smallpox), but
even so it is clear that the vast majority of the population at

risk were protected either by inoculation, vaccination or a combination of both (this was stated by Forbes). Vaccination was more popular amongst the "upper and middle classes" and inoculation amongst "paupers" and others "of the same class of society". Forbes does not say much about the practice of inoculation at the beginning of the nineteenth century, except that "the last general inoculation . . . was in 1806", which implies that it was the last of a preceding series. This is confirmed by the claims of one of the amateur inoculators practising in 1821— Pearce, a farmer—who had practised during the earlier period, and as we have seen boasted "that of 10,000 persons inoculated by his father, not one died, and that his own success has been as great." Pearce also claimed that his mother had been a very successful inoculator, which was not unusual in this area, for Forbes noted "many sly poachers of the other" sex who were rivals to Pearce; he also had three male rivals who were amateur inoculators—a knife-grinder, a fishmonger, and a whitesmith.[320]

From the evidence about the practice of inoculation during the period that vaccination began to be practised, we may conclude that inoculation was almost universally established before the introduction of vaccination, except in large towns such as London, Manchester, Glasgow, Newcastle and Whitehaven—in these latter places vaccination was introduced at an early date and on a wide scale, which suggests that inoculation never really became popular in them at any time.[321] It must not be forgotten that only about a fifth of the total population lived in towns of 10,000 and above in 1801,[322] and that in some of them (such as Carlisle, Leeds and London) inoculation had made considerable headway by the end of the eighteenth century. Rowley, a surgeon, in a defence of inoculation published in 1805, claimed that "Small-pox inoculation was a well-known, proved, and absolute prevention from receiving the natural Small-pox infection, as millions of people now living can testify",[323] a conclusion which perhaps is not unjustified in the light of available evidence. Inoculation was eventually abolished by law in 1840, by which time the importance of repeated vaccination had been well established, so diminishing the major objection to it (a limited period of protection). However, even as late as 1840 the Bishop of London could say during the debate of the bill banning inoculation that

"it was well known that, in agricultural districts of the country, there had not been for many years past the least difficulty in obtaining vaccination gratuitously, but many of the ignorant poor were strongly prejudiced against it, and paid a much greater attention to empirics than to the advice of the clergy. He thought that the bill would not do half the good that was intended, unless those persons were prevented, by penalty from practising inoculation."[324]

To understand how the poor and the population at large became so attached to inoculation, and to see the exact extent of inoculation, we must turn to a consideration of the practice of general inoculations, which laid the foundation for the virtual elimination of smallpox.

CHAPTER 5

General Inoculations

The practice of the general inoculation of all vulnerable members of a particular community arose through the interaction of two factors: (*i*) the fear that partial inoculations of only some members of the community would spread the natural form of the disease to the rest; (*ii*) the highly successful innovation of method brought about by the Suttons, which made inoculation both sufficiently safe and cheap to obtain general acceptance. The "airing" of patients and sending them into the community as a part of the Suttons' "cold treatment", aggravated the fears of the vulnerable population, which initially provoked great hostility, but later led to the widespread acceptance of general inoculation. As Thomas Davies the bailiff to the Glynde estate wrote in 1767, the danger of natural smallpox "together with the great Success and liberty of moving about and freedom from even Sickness, in the new method, to all Ages and Constitutions, made me wish I could persuade our little Parish to do as Tunbridge Wells and Ryegate and such places have done *i.e.* to inoculate all in order to be clear of it in about a fortnight or three weeks." Thus ironically, what has traditionally been thought of as a major reason for rejecting inoculation as a cause of falling smallpox mortality—that it spread the natural form of the disease to vulnerable members of the population—was in fact one of the major reasons for the establishment of its near universal practice, with a consequent dramatic impact on mortality.

General inoculation was therefore a logical outgrowth of contemporary belief and practice, although not all parish authorities agreed in the earlier period to find the sums of money required to pay for such relatively large numbers of inoculations. The person whose name and authority came to be most closely associated with the advocacy of general inoculations, was Thomas Dimsdale, who was the most influential single inoculator after Daniel Sutton. The overall history of general inoculations may be largely traced through Dimsdale's writings, and we can start by quoting his account of the success in clearing his home town, Hertford, of smallpox in the period 1766-1774:

"In a former publication, I gave an account of the occasion of a general Inoculation [in 1766] at this place [Hertford]; from that time the town was released from any apprehensions of the disease, until the year 1770, when it appeared again . . . we had then upwards of two hundred and fifty [inoculated] patients, some of whom were new inhabitants, but the rest consisted for the most part of very young children . . . In the year 1774 the disease appeared a third time;

the same request was renewed, and with the same assistance afforded, the whole town was inoculated once more, and now the number amounted only to about 120; from that time we have heard nothing of Small-Pox, and I verily believe, that within these ten years not six persons have died in Hertford of this disease . . ."[325]

Practically all the population at risk must have been inoculated in Hertford, as only about six persons had died from the disease in the previous ten years, and some of these six must have been among the "two or three" which died in 1770 (and presumably in 1774) before the general inoculation took place. Dimsdale contrasted the success of inoculation in Hertford, with what he considered to be the unsatisfactory "partial" inoculation of the town of Bedford:

". . . the melancholy account of the consequences of a precipitate Inoculation of the greatest part of the inhabitants in a populous town [Bedford], within this last year [1778]. A pretty general Inoculation was suddenly agreed on, and within one week 1,100 were inoculated . . . but many others in the same town, from religious opinions, ill health, or timidity could not be prevailed on to assent to the scheme; 250 of these soon caught it, and the distemper proved uncommonly fatal to them, for about two in seven died, so that in a few weeks 59 at least lost their lives from this circumstance."[326]

Dimsdale considered this mass inoculation to be "precipitate" and "melancholy" in consequence, but although 59 people dying from smallpox was obviously of no small consequence, this should be set against the vast majority of the population being protected against the disease. Dimsdale blamed the deaths of the 59 on the partial nature of the inoculation, but he failed to mention that "a bad kind of natural smallpox had broken out in the town before the inoculation began."[327] The actual facts of the situation are not important however from the point of view of the growth of general inoculation; Dimsdale and many contemporaries believed that inoculation was highly contagious, and this was enough to provoke them to insist that all vulnerable members of a community should either be inoculated or removed from the scene where the inoculations were taking place.

Dimsdale published in 1781 what he considered to be the ideal plan of general inoculation and how it should be carried out:

"A list of the names and ages of such inhabitants of every town and village as have not had the small-pox, is first necessary to be obtained; and marks should be made against the names of those, who, on account of their ill state of health, or other reasons, are not thought fit subjects for the operation, in the judgment of the inoculator, and such persons should be provided with a separate abode, where they may not be in danger of receiving the infection: the rest should be collected in one place, inoculated at one time . . . During the whole of this time, and indeed throughout the whole process, the sick may continue at their own houses."[328]

Dimsdale had in effect carried out this plan in Hertford, virtually eliminating smallpox as a result, and extended it to a number of other neighbouring parishes at about the same time; in 1776 he described how the practice of general inoculation had spread:

"Assisted by my learned friend Dr. Ingenhouz and my two sons, I inoculated, at different times, the neighbouring [to Hertford] parishes of East Berkhamstead, Hertingfordbury, Bayford, and the liberty of Brickenden . . . more than 600 [people] . . . this mode of practice, as I have been informed, has been also used successfully by many others in different parts of England. So far as has come to my knowledge, general Inoculations have hitherto been confined to small towns and villages . . ."[329]

Two years later in 1778, Dimsdale noted even further development of general inoculation in the counties surrounding London —he was discussing an expected decline of smallpox deaths in London as a result of country migrants being inoculated before moving to London:

". . . the extensive practice of general Inoculations in the country, which have prevailed in a remarkable manner within the last two years in the counties of Bedford, Bucks, Herts, and Cambridge, and others contiguous to London, and these patients have been generally such inferior persons as may be supposed to supply London. To such extent has this practice been carried, that I imagine the number must amount to many thousands, and for the most part it has been conducted properly, that is to say, every one has been inoculated, or retired from the scene of infection . . ."[330]

This development occurred throughout all areas of the country; Haygarth noted in 1785 that "whole villages in the neighbourhood [Chester], and many other parts of Britain, have been inoculated with one consent",[331] and as we have already seen, Howlett stated earlier in 1781 that when Smallpox appeared in provincial towns and villages "inoculation takes place amongst all ranks of people, the rich and poor, from either choice or necessity, almost instantly have recourse to it."[332]

Once a community had experienced one successful general inoculation, it appears to have become a regular occurrence whenever a smallpox epidemic threatened. Maldon in Essex was one of the first places to undergo a general inoculation—Sutton had inoculated all vulnerable people in the town and had completely cleared it of smallpox in 1764 as we have seen—and general inoculations were subsequently repeated in 1767, 1779, 1788, 1797 and 1806.[333] It is not known exactly how many people were inoculated at any of these dates (except 1764), and the references are merely summary statements, so that, for example, the Maldon parish register merely states on February 17th, 1797—"a General Inoculation/Small-Pox", and on February 27th, 1806— "Small Pox a General Inoculation". It is clear, however, that inoculation was practised quite generally about every nine years, presumably when a new epidemic threatened. By the last two decades of the eighteenth century, the term general inoculation had become so commonplace that it was used in a matter-of-fact way; for example, Jenner quoted a letter from Dr John Earle, stating how "in March 1784, a general inoculation took place at Arlingham" in Gloucestershire,[334] and Jenner himself quite casually referred in his Inquiry to "a general inoculation taking place" in Berkeley in April 1795.[335] Jenner was not the only member of his family to practice smallpox inoculation; "the paupers of the village of Tortworth, in this county (Gloucestershire), were inoculated by Mr Henry Jenner, Surgeon, of Berkeley, in the year 1795,"[336] and G. C. Jenner published "an account of a general inoculation at Painswick (Gloucestershire)" which took place between the end of May and the end of July 1785, seven hundred and thirty-eight people being inoculated.[337] This latter general inoculation was only resorted to after the outbreak of a virulent smallpox epidemic, which "destroyed nearly one-third of those who were infected by it."[338] This delay in resorting to inoculation until an epidemic had broken out, obviously led to the risk that some of the inoculated would have caught the natural disease before they had time to be protected—and any deaths resulting would be set down as being a result of the inoculation.

Sometimes a parish acted with very great speed when an epidemic threatened. The following is an account of the reaction of the Northwold (in Norfolk) parish authorities taken from the churchwardens accounts:

"Northwold. Jan 28th 1788. At a Meeting of the principal inhabitants of this parish holden at ye Bull Inn, it appered that Ann Robinson a poor widow and her family were Ill with the small pox in the naturell way: that upwards of three hundred and seventy persons legaly setlled who were never had been infected by the small pox where resident in the parish. It was therefore resolved that a genereld innoculation of such uninfected persons should take place . . ."[339]

As most of these 370 people "were unabel to Defray the nessery Expence" of inoculating themselves and their families, the parish paid for the major part of them; 226 were inoculated at the parish expense, 74 paid for it privately.[340] The parish seems to have excluded the poor who had not a legal settlement from this form of medical relief; how common this kind of exclusion was is unknown—it is the only example that has come to light in the evidence reviewed for this book.

Reluctance to undertake a general inoculation could however take extreme forms, and the following instance in Lewes, Sussex for the year 1794 is quoted at some length as it illustrates so vividly both the great fear that smallpox created in people, and the measures and lengths that they were sometimes prepared to go to, in order to contain the spread of the disease and avoid the necessity of a general inoculation:

"On Monday 4th of January, it was represented to the Chief Officers of the Borough that the Small Pox was at that time at its full height in the House of George Apted, in St. Mary's Lane . . . he was determined they [his family] should all remain where they were. The Constables then resorted to the early Measures they saw within their Power; they caused a high wood Fence to be erected around his Door, and placed a Watch both by Night and Day, to prevent the infected Family from mixing any more with other Persons in the Neighbourhood. On Friday the 10th at Six in the Evening, another Meeting on the same Business was called by the Constables. At this second Meeting (which entirely filled the Town Hall) it appeared that the Disorder further manifested itself in the families of several other Persons within the said St. Mary's Lane, and that each of them refused to remove, the Determination of this Meeting was to block up the infected Lane at both Ends . . . Several of the Heads of infected Families having, in the Hall (at a meeting on Saturday, 11th), refused to remove their Children etc or to suffer them to be removed, a general Inoculation was by some thought advisable; it was therefore deemed proper to request the Constables again to adjourn the Meeting to the next Evening (Sunday) and to give the most public Notice by Hand Bills and by Proclamation at the several Parish Churches that the Question of the Necessity of a General Inoculation would on that Evening, be discussed and determined . . . It was afterwards resolved that in the Consequence of the Opinions given to the Faculty, a General

Inoculation **does not** at present appear necessary. On Monday, the 13th every Gentleman of the Faculty within the Borough with one of the Constables visited the infected Families, and finding the Disorder much wider spread than they had expected, they desired the Constables again to call a Meeting of the Inhabitants which was very numerously and respectably attended—at this Meeting it was determined that a General Inoculation being an Evil much less dreaded than a General Infection, in the Natural Way, which was very likely to take Place within this Town & Neighbourhood, it was solemnly put and carried that 'Circumstances as are at present are, a GENERAL INOCULATION ought to be adopted within the Borough': The Inoculation accordingly commenced the next Day, & was continued till the 20th when the Town was again convened, & determined that the General Inoculation in the Town of Lewes, ought to Cease, and that a Continuance thereof, by the Introduction of Strangers, would be injurious to the Trade etc of the Gentlemen who had undertaken the Business by Inoculation to desist from that Practice within the said Borough. The number of Persons inoculated in Consequence of the above mentioned Resolutions ammounted according to the best Accounts the Constables could produce to about 2890, of which number 46 died under Inoculation.

John Richards
Arthur Lee.
(Constables)."[341]

This account reveals a great deal about contemporary attitudes to smallpox and inoculation. Ironically, the reluctance to resort to general inoculation was a part of a self-fulfilling prophecy; 46 of the 2,890 people inoculated died—and probably the majority of these deaths were the result of previous infection with natural smallpox during the period of delay. These deaths would have fuelled the fear of the next general inoculation, and the circular process would continue. However, in spite of this marring of the effectiveness of the general inoculation, it was in overall terms a great success. Given that about one in three people catching smallpox died of the disease at this time, the number of lives saved was dramatic (it would be of the order of 950 people); the extent of the inoculation is indicated by the fact that the total population of the town of Lewes was only 4,909 in 1801—thus well over half of the population would have been inoculated in 1794.

The number of people dying from smallpox caught during the delay before general inoculation seems to have varied greatly from place to place. I have already referred to the advertisements placed by the Ewell authorities in the *Gentleman's*

Magazine describes a mass inoculation without loss of life and that entered by the Overseers of Irthlingborough in the *Northampton Mercury*, giving an account of the "upwards of Five Hundred People" inoculated in the village without a death in 1778; a similar entry was placed in the *Ipswich Journal* by the minister, surgeons and churchwardens of the town of Diss in Norfolk on the 3rd June, 1784:

"In March last, the small-pox broke out in this town; it was of so favourable a kind, that the sick did not confine themselves to their houses; by means of which the disease was communicated to several families, which induced the inhabitants to submit to a general inoculation. In Eight or Nine days, more than Eleven hundred were inoculated, from the age of one month to between Eighty and Ninety years; of which number not One person died. Scarce any of the poor were kept from their labour more than Two or Three days; many not at all. These circumstances are published as inducement to other parishes to adopt the same happy means of irradicating this dreadful disorder."[342]

The motives of the parish authorities may not have been as unambiguously altruistic as claimed, for the advertisement was prefaced with the statement that "there is not ONE PERSON in This Town that has the SMALL POX", and there are reasons to believe that trade may have been a factor in informing the public of this fact. We saw how in Lewes the town authorities were anxious to suppress inoculation once the general inoculation of the townsfolk was over, because it would be "injurous to the Trade" of the town—people fearing to come into a town where smallpox, even in the inoculated form, was known to be present—and this motive to preserve trade provoked other parish authorities to place protective advertisements in their local newspaper, e.g. the churchwardens, overseers, physician and surgeons of the parish of Hadleigh in Suffolk put the following entry in the *Ipswich Journal* for June 17th, 1778:

"Whereas a general Inoculation for the Small Pox took place in this parish in the month of March last. We, whose names are hereunder written, do hereby give notice, That the said town is now, and has for some time past been, entirely FREE from the said infection, and that the parish may be resorted to with safety."[343]

The clearing of a market town of smallpox must have been a very great economic incentive for parish authorities to pay for general inoculations; smallpox was often in market towns for periods of up to two years in the pre-inoculation era, and this could virtually ruin the trade of a town for that period.

The economics of inoculation is brought out most clearly in the following very detailed account of a general inoculation carried out at Brighton in 1786; it seems to have been conducted along the lines suggested by Dimsdale, with a house-to-house survey of all those who had smallpox previously, and those still vulnerable to the disease. I quote the account in full, as it is unrivalled in the detail that it supplies about a specific general inoculation:

"TOWN OF BRIGHTHELMSTON
      Be it Remembered that on the 25 Day of Jany 1786 at a Public Vestry held at the Town Hall in Brighthelmston Pursuant to Public Notice given, It was (in consequence of the Heavy Expense Brought on the said Town by the Removal of Patients in the Natural Small Pox to the Neighbouring Pest Houses, which usually amounted to Six Pounds Each Person and in consideration of the Small Pox Breaking out in Several Different Places in the Town at once) then Unanimously Agreed by the Inhabitants there assembled that no more Persons should be Removed at the Parish Expense. And it also appearing Impossible to Prevent the Infection from Becoming General It was also Agreed for the Poor in the Town House and such other of the Inhabitants of said Town to be inoculated as should be Deemed Proper objects of Relief, by the Churchwardens, Overseers, and Twelve of the Principal Inhabitants of said Town Appointed by the Vestry as a Committee for managing and conducting Inoculating the above Poor at the Parish Expense.
      And for carrying the foregoing into Execution in the most Exact Manner it was Determined to find out the Numbers of Persons who Had the Small Pox and those who Had Not had the same in said Town—
      And on a Survey Made by the above Committee and Parish Officers Were Found the Following Numbers

Jany 26 1786	Numbers who Had	Numbers Not Had
In West Street etc.	351	322
In Middle Do & Lanes	231	272
North Street & Do	234	295
Ship & Black Lyon Do	318	336
Knab Cliff Bn Place	260	291
Little East Street		
East Street N. Row	308	291
Steyne & Pool Lane		
Poor in the House	31	50
Numbers Supposed to be Got into Town after Taking Numbers	—	30
	1,733	1,887

Out of the Above Number Five Hundred and forty five were Inoculated at the Parish Expense.

At the Same Vestry Messrs Lowdell Gilbert, Parkhurst & Tilson Surgeons and Apothecaries of This Town Agreed to Inoculate all the Poor Above mentioned, all Servants and Day Labourers at Half a Crown Each, Medicines Included—and all Other Persons at three Half Crowns Each.

In consequence of the Foregoing the Inoculation Commenced on the 27 of Jany and in Course of a few Day's the Aforesaid Numbers of Eighteen Hundred Eighty Seven were Inoculated—Persons of all ages from One Day to Near Fourscore Years Old.

It Also Appears that by the Goodness of Providence and the Care and Attendance of the Physical Gentn though in the above Number were Persons of all Ages and Complaints Women very Near their time etc. Yet the very Small Number of [blank] were all that Died of the Small Pox.

The Expense of Attending Patients

1785	Fifteen in Natural Small Pox to Dr. Lander Dennett Carr etc.	£ 82 16 0
1736	Ten Natural Patients & Expense of carrying them Also Funerals of Two at Mr Dennett	£ 57 4 4
		£140 0 4
1786	Expense of Inoculating 545 Persons a 2/6 ea	£ 68 2 6
	To Expense of Relief to Different Families By flour Coals Cash etc. During their Inoculations	£ 82 17 6
		£151 0 0

Messrs. Dennett of Storrington and Sanders of the Broyle assisted in the General Inoculation of the Town and Had a Considerable Number of Patients on Same Plan as the Doctors of the Town."[344]

The cost of nursing and burying twenty-five natural smallpox patients was nearly as great as the inoculation of 545 poor people in the town. Economic considerations were listed even before the threat of a smallpox epidemic as factors in bringing about the general inoculation, which appears to have been carried out with great thoroughness. All of the 1,887 people not yet protected against smallpox were inoculated, although only 545 of these were paid for by the parish (the large total numbers involved may have accounted for this low proportion). The general inoculation was obviously highly successful, although according to a local historian writing in 1818, 34 of the 1,887 cases died; a general inoculation was organised along the same lines six years later in 1794, and the enumeration of the population revealed a greatly increased total of 5,669—of which 2,113 were inoculated (about 250 coming in from neighbouring villages).[345] "No more than 50 died" of the 2,113 inoculated, but it is likely that in both the 1786 and 1794 general inoculations, the delay in starting inoculation before a number of natural smallpox cases had occurred, contributed very heavily to deaths amongst the inoculated. However, it would seem that only a very small proportion of the total inoculated were affected in this way; perhaps a more typical general inoculation was that which occurred at Tenterden, Kent in 1798, when "toward the end of the year there was a general Inoculation took place and out of eleven hundred and sixty seven who had the complaint only three died."[346]

Most general inoculations seem to have included people in all age groups, ranging in Brighton in 1786 "from One Day to Near Fourscore Years." Similarly at Dursley in Gloucestershire when the local surgeon, Mr Fry, undertook a general inoculation in the Spring of 1797, he "inoculated fourteen hundred and seventy-five patients, of all ages, from a fortnight old to seventy years."[347] However, with the repetition of general inoculations every few years when epidemics threatened, the average age of those inoculated obviously dropped significantly; for example, Mr Wayte a surgeon who practised at Calne in Wiltshire described the general inoculation of the parish as follows:

"in September, 1793, when the poor of the parish were inoculated . . . we inoculated six hundred and upwards . . . Besides the poor, I inoculated about two hundred [private] patients . . . Now in inoculating a whole parish, we have no choice of patients, all ages, and the sickly as well as others, were inoculated, but these were mostly children, as I assisted in inoculating the whole parish, about twelve or thirteen years ago."[348]

There were only eight deaths registered as being due to smallpox in Calne during the period 1783-1802, and as we shall in a later chapter, repeated general inoculations led to the inevitable consequence: the almost total elimination of smallpox.

CHAPTER 6

The Practice of Inoculation in America, Scotland, Ireland and on the Continent of Europe

It is possible to discuss the practice of inoculation in other countries in the European orbit only very briefly, but having attempted to re-define the nature and effectiveness of inoculation, it might be of some interest to look at some of the evidence on its practice in these countries. One general point can be made at the outset: those countries where smallpox tended to return only infrequently and therefore take the form of dramatic epidemics, were usually the ones where inoculation was most widely practised. This was true of the British American Colonies (later the United States), Ireland and the Highland areas of Scotland; I have discussed earlier the psychology associated with the epidemiology of the endemic as against the epidemic form of the disease—townspeople tending to become fatalistically resigned to a regularly returning disease affecting only a minority of their children in any one year, country people reacting with great panic at the prospect of an epidemic striking a large proportion of the population at just one point in time.

America is undoubtedly one of the countries in which inoculation was most widely practised, which makes it all the more surprising that no comprehensive scholarly study of its history has ever been published for that country. We have seen in the earlier period how active inoculators were in the American Colonies, and how much influence they had through the publication of the works of people like Boylston and Kilpatrick. The neglect of the history of American inoculation is all the more surprising given the comprehensiveness of some of its statistics; the figures for Boston cover the whole of the eighteenth century period and include details of population, numbers of natural smallpox cases (and deaths), and the number of people inoculated at different times. I shall discuss the complete set of figures in the last chapter; here it is sufficient to note the rapid growth in the practice of inoculation, particularly after 1752, so that by the end of the century all but a tiny minority of the vulnerable population were protected by inoculation. The following Table gives a summary of the relevant figures:

Inoculation in Eighteenth Century Boston, U.S.A.[349]

Date	1721	1730	1752	1764	1776	1788	1792
Natural Smallpox Cases	5759	3600	5545	699	304	122	232
Numbers Inoculated	287	400	2124	4977	4988	2121	9152
Left the Town			1843	1537			262
Escaped Disease in Town			174	519			221

This Table reveals better than other evidence the ability of inoculation to protect against smallpox; by the end of the century in 1792, there were only 232 cases of natural smallpox as against the 9152 people inoculated. Only 262 people chose to leave the town rather than be inoculated, and there were 221 people who stayed in the town but escaped the disease (earlier I pointed out that this was strong evidence against the contagiousness of inoculation). In terms of chronology, it is interesting to note that as in England, there was fairly significant increase in the practice of inoculation at the beginning of the 1750s. In Boston, however, the major growth of inoculation occurred in 1764—before the Suttonian innovation of technique—and although the Suttons had exported their method to Boston through their partnership scheme, the evidence is that popular inoculation arrived before their innovation in technique did. It would appear that an improvement in method had taken place between 1730 and 1752 in Boston—the mortality rate amongst the inoculated dropped from 3.0 per cent to 1.4 per cent[350]—and this may have been associated with the lighter method of inoculation advocated by Ranby, Sloane and Kilpatrick. But this evidence on mortality amongst the inoculated is extremely unreliable as far as Boston is concerned; inoculation was only practised after smallpox had broken out in the town—it was forbidden by law at other times, at least in the later period—and many of the deaths amongst the inoculated were almost certainly due to this delay. This would explain why the mortality rate amongst the inoculated in 1792—2.0 per cent—was about as high as when inoculation was first introduced into the town in 1721 (2.0 per cent).[351] Notwithstanding this mortality amongst the inoculated, we will see later that inoculation very dramatically reduced the total number of deaths from smallpox in Boston.

Although inoculation was introduced into Scotland at about the same time as it was in England, it grew much more slowly in the former place. 5553 persons were known to have been inoculated in Scotland by 1764,[352] which is very much smaller, even taking into account relative sizes of population, than the estimated 200,000 inoculations in England by 1766. Monro, who drew up the account of inoculation in Scotland, summarized the position in 1764 as follows:

"The greater number of the gentry, and most of the medical gentlemen . . . have their children inoculated; but the . . . tempting of Providence, weighs more among many of the populace, who will not allow the small-pox to be artificially implanted."[353]

Calvinist theology again provided arguments for the opponents of inoculation, although from evidence about to be considered it appears that other factors were of greater importance in retarding the spread of inoculation in Scotland. The differential spread of inoculation in Scotland and England was reflected in a statement by Aberdour, an Edinburgh physician, in 1791:

"It is now about seventy years since inoculation was practised in England, and sixty in Scotland, and though it is now become general, still there are many individuals who will not permit inoculation; and many objections are made to the practice, especially by the lower class of people in North Britain [Scotland]."[354]

Fortunately, we are in a position to assess this statement in some detail as far as Scotland is concerned, for many incumbents discussed inoculation in their parishes in their returns compiled for the *Statistical Account of Scotland* during the 1790s.[355] Of the 243 incumbents who discussed inoculation, 162 said it was widely practised in their parishes, as against 91 who said that it had still to become general. Examples will best illustrate this difference. In 1792 the incumbent of Durrinish, Skye, wrote:

"this increase in population may be attributed . . . above all, to the inoculation of the smallpox, which has been universally practised in this island for thirty years past, and has been the means of preserving many lives."[356]

This may be contrasted to Eaglesham where, according to the incumbent in 1792

"the smallpox carry off great numbers of children; but there is no reconciling the minds of the lower ranks to inoculation."[357]

Most incumbents who stated that inoculation was not general in their parishes also attempted to explain why. One recurring explanation given was as follows:

"The notions of absolute predestination, which are still deeply rooted in the minds of the country people, lead the generality of them to look upon inoculation as implying an impious distrust of Divine Providence, and a vain attempt to alter its irreversible decrease."[358]

This religious objection was perhaps a generalisation of a more concrete attitude, that "the thought of bringing trouble on their children as they call it, with their own hands, outweigh every argument that can be advanced in its favour."[359]. This was one of the initial major reasons why parents were reluctant to have their children inoculated in England, and it is of interest to examine why this attitude persisted in Scotland much more than it did in England. The Calvinist religious belief in predestination no doubt buttressed this attitude, but perhaps more important was the age incidence and nature of smallpox epidemics in Scotland. Monro had noted in 1765 that

"The inhabitants of Scotland generally have the smallpox in their infancy or childhood; very few adults being seen here in this disease."[360]

Monro was somewhat puzzled by this, but suggested that it may have amongst other things been due to the fact that "in the villages the peasants are generally assistant to their neighbours of whose family any is sick" and did not "fly from the place where it [smallpox] is" as they did in England.[361] The periodicity of smallpox epidemics was, however, partly a function of the geographical situation of a place and areas such as the Western Isles are known to have been free from smallpox for very long periods of time. The same was probably true of the Highlands, and it is no accident that variolation was almost universally practised in such areas; for example, the incumbent of Portingal in Perthshire wrote in 1792 "that fewer children die in the Highlands than almost anywhere, particularly since inoculation has been universally practised, which it has been, for a good many years back, to the saving of many lives."[362] Areas where epidemics were infrequent were likely to respond in panic to the threat of an epidemic (as they did in England), and perhaps this was the most important factor in determining the rate of spread of inoculation in different parts of Scotland. However, several incumbents noted that even in the areas where inoculation was not general, "the people entertain no prejudice against inoculation, but grudge the expense of it."[363] Unlike England, there was no organised system of poor relief at the parish level which could have been used for free inoculation of the poor, although Sinclair claimed that this problem was overcome in large measure through charitable inoculation paid for by the local gentry, free inoculation by the medical profession and even the practice of inoculation by ministers of the Church. I have already indicated the extent of inoculation during the 1790s—162 of 243 ministers saying it was generally practised in their parishes. The relative lag of inoculation in Scotland compared to England was reflected in the acceptance of vaccination in Scotland:

"it [vaccination in Edinburgh] has been much more generally adopted by the lower orders of the People, than ever the inoculation for the Small Pox, and they [the Royal College of Physicians of Edinburgh] believe the same to obtain all over Scotland."[364]

Some parents still objected "to the production of any disease among their children", but it appears that vaccination was more popular in Scotland than in England during this period, indirectly confirming the conclusion that inoculation was less general in the former than in the latter by the end of the eighteenth century.

Inoculation was introduced into Ireland in 1725 but was only very sporadically practised until the advent of the Suttonian method. Little is known of the exact chronology of its spread. We have seen previously that the Suttons appointed several partners in different parts of Ireland, and Houlton noted in 1768 that of the imitators of the Suttons, "some, I am informed since my arrival in Ireland, are now travelling over several parts of the kingdom . . . ."[365] This probably was the beginning of the practice of itinerant inoculation in Ireland which was to become very important. There were very few hospitals or doctors in Ireland at this time, and this was related to the vast majority of the Irish population living in isolated hamlets and scattered cabins.[366] Some inoculations were performed by county infirmaries,[367] but most were performed by "individuals [who] proceed from village to village several times during the year for the purpose of inoculating the infantile population."[368] We are fortunate to have a detailed description of one of these itinerant inoculators; a Frenchman, De Latocnaye, gave the following account of a meeting which took place during the period 1796-97:

"In the mountains (of Mayo) I fell in with a man who had the air of being something of a *bon-vivant*. He told me that his profession was that of an inoculator, and that he was about to inoculate the children of the peasantry in this wild country. He assured me positively that of 361 children inoculated by him this year only one died. When it is understood that if he has been unfortunate enough to have a child die on his hands, not only is he not paid, but he must escape promptly in order to avoid a beating by the afflicted parents, it will be seen that the poor devil must take great pains with his patients. But for the death of his patron, the inoculator, who was born in the area, would have become a priest. It was just the time when inoculation had begun to be put into practice and the terrible effects often produced by smallpox on these mountain folk gave him the idea of visiting them and taking up the profession of inoculator, after he had taken some lessons in the hospitals. Now he has practising with success for thirty or forty years, but all he makes by way of income is not more than thirty or forty pounds sterling per annum. On the Continent, not only would the peasants refuse to allow their children to be inoculated, but even people comfortably off would make a like refusal. In England well-meaning proprietors are often obliged to beg the parents to submit; in Scotland they have not yet succeeded in securing the adoption of the method, and yet it is generally adopted in Ireland even in its wildest parts."[369]

There may have been a note of exaggeration in some of De Latocnaye's statements—we have just seen that inoculation was widely practised in some parts of Scotland—but the overall emphasis on the universality of the practice in Ireland (and its almost total neglect on the Continent), was almost certainly correct. James Moore, the first director of the National Vaccine Establishment, agreed with De Latocnaye's conclusions while trying to explain why the Irish were so reluctant to accept vaccination:

"Variolous inoculation was formerly patronized in Ireland by the Popish Clergy, and had, therefore, been much more generally adopted by the common people, than in any other country. The degree of security which this afforded, rendered many unwilling to try a new plan . . . "[370]

The emphasis on the importance of religious influence was probably misplaced; while it may have been a factor in the popularity of inoculation in Ireland, the most important variable was almost certainly an epidemiological one: the remoteness of most Irish communities, and thus the highly epidemic and dramatic nature of smallpox when it struck a particular area.

The resistance of the Irish to vaccination led to a number of accounts—both current and retrospective—of the activities of the inoculators. For example, one opponent of inoculation described in 1807 itinerant inoculators as follows:

"Variolous Inoculation had been long, almost exclusively, in the hands of a particular branch of the profession, whose prejudices and interests were strongly opposed to the new practice [of vaccination]; and by their being the usual medical attendants in families, and especially in the diseases of children, their opinions had greater effect upon the minds of parents."[371]

These inoculators were elsewhere described [in 1807] in more pejorative terms as "the lower class of apothecaries", "Quacks travelling about the country" and "some Quacks and old women."[372] It appears that the apothecaries concentrated on the towns and the "Itinerant Quacks" on the countryside. This was not all that dissimilar to England during the same period (1807), except that the "empiric" inoculators in Ireland were necessarily itinerant. It is clear that inoculation was very extensively practised in Ireland, for as the Royal Dublin College of Physicians reported in 1807:

> "The Small Pox is rendered a much less formidable disease in this country by the frequency of Inoculation for it . . . hence parents, not unnaturally, objected to the introduction of a new disease [vaccination], rather than not recur to that [inoculation], with the mildness and safety of which they were well acquainted."[373]

This conclusion is confirmed by other independent evidence; the Rev. H. Townsend described in his *Statistical Survey of the County of Cork* published in 1810, "the universal custom of inoculating children for the smallpox."[374] Although there is no information about the chronology of the spread of inoculation between 1768 and 1807, it appears from remarks made on the subject in the latter year it had been practised for some considerable time, e.g. Dr Castle wrote from the area of Derry in 1807:

> "And it is remarkable that altho' this latter inoculation [vaccination] is but sparingly practised in the neighbouring country, the former variolous inoculation is not followed as much as it was won't to be amongst the country folks a few years ago . . . "[375]

The earlier practice of inoculation was also suggested by the previously quoted remark, "Variolous Inoculation had been long, almost exclusively, in the hands" of itinerant inoculators. These inoculators seemed to have practised in all parts of the country, for a summary of all the letters sent to the Royal Dublin College of Physicians in 1807 stated that "Quacks travelling about the country and inoculating with variolous matter . . . are mentioned in the letters which have been received on the subject,"[376] and practically all letters quoted mentioned them. Inoculation continued to be practised in Ireland until at least 1875 (particularly in rural areas), and Sir William Wilde noticed the extensive activities of the inoculators as late as 1851.[377] Ireland like England, was one of the few European countries in which vaccination was not generally practised during the firsty forty or fifty years of the nineteenth century, and members of the Irish medical profession explicitly linked this with the nearly universal practice of inoculation.

Other than the places considered, inoculation appears to have been practised only on a limited scale in Europe; Dimsdale, who had personal experience of inoculation in Continental countries (*e.g.* Russia and Austria) stated in 1778 that "it is extremely probable, more persons of late years have been inoculated here [in England], than in all the rest of Europe."[378] We saw earlier that it was used regularly and extensively in the Hague and at Geneva, but we cannot discuss the practice of variolation on the Continent in any detail, except to point out that it was strongly encouraged in some countries (Sweden, Russia and Austria)[379] and apparently hardly practised at all in others (Spain).[380] The relative lack of popularity of inoculation on the Continent was reflected in the willingness of most of these countries enthusiastically to embrace vaccination, although ironically, vaccination in the earlier part of the nineteenth century was almost certainly only a more attenuated form of the old inoculation.

CHAPTER 7

The Reliability of Smallpox Mortality Registration

The mortality from smallpox is substantially determined by the type of virus responsible for the disease, and as we have already seen, although there were only thought to be two major variants—variola major and variola minor—it now appears that there is a whole spectrum of viruses, ranging from the very mild to the very severe. Smallpox is fairly easily recognizable from its skin lesions and other symptoms with a distinctive chronology in their appearance, although Dixon has pointed out that

> "It cannot be too strongly emphasized that in the 'difficult' case of smallpox the skin lesions may closely resemble those occurring in other diseases, but the timing of their appearance in relation to the general symptoms determines whether the disease can or cannot be smallpox."[361]

Although the timing of the appearance of symptoms enables smallpox to be distinguished from other diseases in which skin lesions occur, it occasionally happens that smallpox is confused with these other diseases, particularly measles and chicken-pox. This type of confusion is illustrated by an account of an unsuccessful inoculation given by Dimsdale:

> ". . . a general inoculation having been performed in a parish in the country . . . they judged themselves, they were safe from any danger from the smallpox—some made the trial, and went into houses where the real smallpox ranged; this trial cost them dear, for I believe most, if not all, fell with the real smallpox, and died. On a strict enquiry it was reported, that the matter used in inoculation was taken from a subject having the chicken-pox."[382]

This type of mistake must have been very rare, for it is the only example that has come to light from an examination of historical records used in this research. The main reason for the ability of contemporaries during the eighteenth century to recognize smallpox was its epidemic nature in most parts of the country, where it returned regularly every few years; under such conditions smallpox must have been very easy to recognise.[383] In large towns, however, it would have been more difficult because of the endemic nature of the disease in such places; for example, in London smallpox deaths were recorded every week during the seventeenth and eighteenth century.[384] In such a situation it would be possible to confuse individual cases of smallpox with other diseases such as measles and chicken-pox.

There is one form of smallpox which has only recently been recognized, as it does not give rise to the eruption of lesions, the main symptom by which smallpox has been historically recognized. It has been labelled Fulminating Smallpox (Purpura Variola), and is of sufficient importance to describe at length. Dixon has given the following account of this form of the disease:

"After an incubation period of about eleven to twelve days the patient is suddenly taken ill, with a feeling of intense prostration accompanied by severe headache, and often backache. In spite of these symptoms the patient is very 'wide awake' and peculiarly apprehensive. In some patients the infection is so overwhelming that death may occur within twenty-four to thirty-six hours with no outward manifestations at all . . . At post-mortem there may be a few haemorrhages in the submucosa, in the respiratory and alimentary tracts and in the heart muscle, the latter possibly contributing to death in some cases. The appearances are very indefinite, with no findings on which to base a certain diagnosis . . . This is "sledgehammer" smallpox, and the diagnosis both clinical and at autopsy is impossible unless smallpox is thought of and unless laboratory facilities are available and used to grow the virus to detect soluble antigen in the blood during life, or after death. If the patient survives more than forty-eight hours there is often a slight but temporary improvement in the general condition, followed by the appearance of an erythema on the face and back of the hands, and a blotchy erythema on the arms and trunk, particularly the anterior abdominal and upper part of the thighs . . . The erythematous areas of the skin will reveal petechial which during the next twenty-four hours rapidly enlarge forming ecchynoses of a peculiar bluish-purple colour . . . but just before death, which occurs within forty-eight hours of the onset of these haemorrhages, the whole body may be affected. When the haemorrhages occur only in the 'bathing drawers' area, a confident diagnosis of smallpox can be made; but when the haemorrhages are more general, as is common, the picture has no completely characteristic features to distinguish it from other hyper-acute infections, although in smallpox there is a greater tendency towards symmetry . . . With the appearance of haemorrhages in the mucous membrane or skin the patient's life may be terminated by massive haematenesis, intestinal or uterine haemorrhage . . . From the diagnostic point of view it cannot be overemphasized that the absence of any vescular eruption is the main feature of this condition and increases the difficulty in differentiating it from other acute haemorrhagic catastrophes. Mortality 100 per cent."[385]

This form of smallpox probably occurs for two major reasons: (1) the virulence of the smallpox virus; (2) the defencelessness, weakness or lack of resistance on the part of the host. It tends to attack most commonly at the extreme ages of life (young infants and old people),[386] and is particularly manifest when smallpox attacks a community which has been free of the disease previously, such as the American Indians, whole tribes of which were wiped out by smallpox during the seventeenth and eighteenth centuries.[387] The vulnerability of the extremes of age is probably due to constitutional weakness, whereas populations such as the American Indians suffered from an absence of genetically acquired resistance to the disease. How does the existence of fulminating smallpox affect this study? Firstly it appears that the haemorrhagic fulminating form was sometimes recognized as smallpox; as early as the seventeenth century, Sydenham recognized the existence of this form of smallpox:

"this summer . . . the pox was in many apt to turn black and there would appear blew spots upon the skin . . . **Purple spots** . . . declare the great malignity . . . with the certainty of the patient's death."[388]

Later, at Kendal and the surrounding area in 1772 there prevailed

"a false species of the smallpox, which has carried off more than 700 people. The affected were at first taken with a very uncommon bleeding at the nose, and generally expired immediately after the first stage of the disorder, which was so putrid in nature, that the whole body of the deceased was covered with large purple blotches, and was exceedingly offensive even before dissolution."[389]

This disease was presumably recognized as smallpox because of the presence of more ordinary forms of smallpox in the area. In other cases, however, fulminating smallpox may have been thought to be another disease. Possibly an example of this is an epidemic which broke out in Norway in 1741:

"It must have been a highly dangerous type of typhus which in some unknown way had gained a foothold in Norway in the autumn of 1741. In a vivid description of the course of the disease, Hanneria described it as 'quite as infectious and fatal as the plague itself'. Death often came with a haemorrhage."[390]

There was certainly an epidemic of smallpox in neighbouring Sweden at the same time, which would tend to confirm our suspicion about the disease in Norway. Although contemporaries noted that a very severe haemorrhagic disease was somehow associated with smallpox, they did not always recognize it as a form of smallpox; Thomas Short writing in 1749 on the history of epidemics in England stated:

"In 1670, 71 and 72 reigned an irregular Small Pox . . . this gave way to the Bloody Flux, and returned again when that was out."[391]

It seems possible that this 'Bloody Flux' was a form of fulminating smallpox, and as the bloody flux was considered a separate disease and registered as such, it is likely that much smallpox mortality arising from the fulminating disease went unrecognized. Some contemporaries were aware of the under-registration of smallpox mortality because of the fulminating nature of the disease amongst very young infants. It was recognized that smallpox killed many young children (particularly under the age of six months) before the usual eruption of pustular lesions, and such deaths were invariably accompanied by convulsive fits; for example, Dr Percival wrote in 1768:

"A considerable number of those who die of the natural disease, before the expulsion of the variolous eruption, are infants or very young children . . . Hence the convulsive paroxysms which often precede the appearance of the pustules . . . are always alarming, and when they happen to very young infants are frequently fatal."[392]

This conclusion about the effects of smallpox on young infants was confirmed by the experience of inoculating the same age group; one of the deaths of the inoculated cases enumerated by Jurin during the 1720s was "Adam Urquart, Son of William Urquart, Esq., of Meldrum aged One Year and a half, [who] was inoculated at Meldrum in Aberdeenshire, August 29, 1726, sicken'd the Seventh Day, and died the Eighth Day before any Appearance of an Eruption, of Fits . . ."[393] Most deaths from smallpox without regular pustular eruptions and accompanied by convulsive fits appear to have occurred amongst infants under the age of five months. Monro in his account of inoculation in Scotland described the effects of inoculation amongst children and the importance of the age of the child:

"Several, considering how much more liable very young children are to convulsions (the most frequent dangerous symptom in the inoculated smallpox) than those farther advanced in life, decline performing inoculation in very young infants . . . More of the patients who died of inoculation were killed by convulsions, near the time of eruption of pimples, or upon their subsiding on the second or third day after their first appearance, and by erysipelatous or rashy eruptions, with spasms when the small-pox were blackening, than by any other cause . . . Of twelve infants, inoculated within a fortnight of their birth, not one had the small-pox; but in some of them a rash appeared about the time when the variolous eruption uses to be seen—Children five months old, inoculated at the same time, and with matter from the same subject, had the smallpox in the regular manner."[394]

The implication of Monro's description is that the majority of the inoculated died under the age of five months from a form of smallpox which may have been of the fulminating type. There are other descriptions of deaths of inoculated infants which confirm this interpretation,[395] but with the onset of post-Suttonian inoculation these become difficult to find as the much safer method of inoculation led to very few deaths even amongst infants. Although the existence of large numbers of deaths from smallpox amongst young infants was frequently noted by contemporary medical writers, this recognition did not necessarily lead to registration unless accompanied by the classical symptoms of smallpox. Haygarth pointed out that

"The disease most fatal to infants is convulsions, arising from various causes; one of them is the small-pox. The two circumstances will explain the reason why, under one year old, the proportion of deaths by the small-pox is less than in subsequent periods . . ."[306]

This conclusion is confirmed by the available statistical evidence on smallpox mortality amongst different age groups of young children during the eighteenth century:

Number of Children dying from Smallpox at different Ages

	0-5 months	6-11 months	1-2 years
Manchester, 1768-1774[397]	21	119	226
Warrington, 1773[398]	8	39	84
Chester, 1774[399]	7	44	38
London, 1774-1796[400]	6	18	44

There were very few infants under the age of six months dying from smallpox and one possible explanation is the non-registration of smallpox deaths due to the fulminating form of the disease amongst this group. Another explanation, for which there is good evidence, is that infants are born with a form of natural immunity—the exact nature of which is unknown[401]—which protects them from attack by smallpox for four or five months after birth until this immunity declines with age. In spite of this type of natural immunity, it appears from evidence considered in a number of places in this book, that infants over the age of two weeks were often successfully inoculated, although it was recognized by contemporaries that this was a little hazardous on account of the danger of the complications such as convulsions and the like. Probably both explanations discussed are relevant to infant deaths: the naturally acquired immunity at birth protected against **attack** from smallpox in many cases, but where the disease managed to penetrate this immunity barrier— either through inoculation or the forms of natural attack described by Percival—it struck in a fulminating manner, producing convulsions and the rapid onset of death. Most of these fulminating infant deaths probably were not registered as being due to smallpox, and this must have been a considerable factor in the under-registration of smallpox deaths in large towns like London where the disease was endemic and therefore struck particularly at young children. It would have been much less important in the countryside where smallpox was an epidemic disease returning every few years, therefore affecting adults as well as children. In Godalming, Surrey for example, where epidemics returned about every thirteen years, of a total of 157 deaths from smallpox during the period 1701-23, 76 were of adults.[402] Only a minority of the total population lived in large towns in England during the eighteenth century, so it might be thought that the under-registration of infants' deaths from smallpox is of only minor importance in the context of the wider study. Unfortunately most records of smallpox mortality are for large towns—smaller towns and villages having no system of registration except for parish registers. The under-registration of infants' deaths from smallpox in the large towns is a major source of total under-registration of smallpox mortality. Lettsom estimated that smallpox mortality in London was twice that recorded in the Bills of Mortality, "the generic article 'convulsions' having swallowed up, in his opinion, a large number of the smallpox deaths of infants."[403] Smallpox deaths amongst infants also appear to have been registered under other headings, such as "infants", "chrysoms" and even diarrhoea.[404] It is impossible to know what proportion of smallpox deaths amongst young infants were registered under other headings. Perhaps Lettsom's estimate is as good as any, for he had a great knowledge of the disease of the poor through his work with the *London Dispensary* and the *Society for General Inoculation of the Poor*—in about 1776 he claimed that "during the last three years, I have attended nearly six thousand poor persons, into many of whose habitations I have entered."[405] Whatever the exact degree of under-registration of smallpox mortality due to its registration under other headings for infants, it is a significant factor to be borne in mind when the records of smallpox mortality in large towns are later discussed.

There is one general problem in attempting to estimate the contribution of any one disease to total mortality, and that is the indirect mortality which cannot be specifically attributed to that disease. Peter Newman in his study *Malaria Eradication and Population Growth* concluded that "deaths actually reported as due to malaria constituted only about one-fifth of all those which would have occurred if malaria had not been present."[406] He reached this conclusion by comparing regions in which malaria had been eradicated with those in which there had been little attempt to deal with the disease. This kind of analysis is only possible where there are good statistics of mortality (both total and from specific diseases) in different types of region, and even where this type of data is available, its interpretation often becomes problematical (there has been considerable dispute about the validity of Newman's conclusions). Also, it is not possible to analyze smallpox mortality during the eighteenth century in this way as the relevant statistics are not available. Although Newman's method of analyzing the contribution of a specific disease to total mortality is not applicable to our problem, his findings at least suggest that the indirect mortality arising from a disease can be very significant. In fact this conclusion was reached by some contemporary commentators on smallpox mortality. Jurin wrote in 1724 that it was "notorious that this Distemper [smallpox] frequently occasions other Diseases, of which the Patients die of a considerable Time after."[407] Similarly Lettsom noted over fifty years later in 1778:

". . . there is reason to believe that nearly double the number die annually in the metropolis of the Natural Small-Pox, more than the bills of mortality ascertain . . . some have been deprived of sight; many have been afflicted with the evil and scrophulous complaints, to which they had been previously strangers; many have been disabled in their limbs . . . and more still have languished under hectic symptoms, and at length, emaciated and totally debilitated, they have sunk under their miseries, and filled up the amazing list of consumptions, many of which originated from the violence of the Natural Small-Pox."[408]

It is impossible to assess Lettsom's estimate of the indirect consequences of smallpox, and again we can only note that he had very extensive experience of treating diseases in London, and that his conclusions appear to have been universally accepted by his contemporaries; for example, Watts quoted the following conclusion in his pamphlet on inoculation published in 1767:

"After the distemper [smallpox] is over, there follow inflammations of the eyes, foul ulcers, abscesses, swelling of the joints, pulmonary consumptions, decays and the like."[409]

Similarly, Willan wrote in 1800 of the "glandular swellings, ulcers, cutaneous affections, disease of the lungs" which followed smallpox.[410] Although most of these secondary complications would have affected mortality indirectly, it does appear that delayed death from smallpox was occasionally recognized in the registration of smallpox mortality; in the list of people dying from smallpox in Godalming, Surrey:

> "early in ye Morning Dyed Lawrence Kern's wife of Ffarnecomb after a longe illness when ye smallpox was off from her but was not well after it till she dyed."[411]

Modern scientific studies of secondary diseases arising out of smallpox confirm in overall terms the conclusions of Lettsom and other eighteenth century doctors who wrote on the subject, although because these studies are based on clinical and post-mortem findings, they are unable to provide any statistical measure of the effects of these illnesses on mortality. Dixon has listed the following as secondary causes of death: (a) bronchopneumonia; (b) streptococcal septicaemia; (c) staphlococcal septicemia; (d) pyaemia; (e) multiple staphylococcal abscesses; (f) osteo-myelitis; (g) empyaema.[412] Many of these illnesses of course arise through environmental conditions, particularly poor hygiene, and this would have been a more severe problem in the pre-antibiotic era. By far the most serious of the secondary infections appears to have been broncho-pneumonia; Councilman and his colleagues published their findings in 1909 on the autopsy of fifty-four victims of smallpox as follows:

> "Some degree of bronchitis and broncho-pneumonia was found in fifty-four cases. It did not differ from the forms of broncho-pneumonia so commonly seen in diptheria . . . These lung lesions were found in all stages of the disease, from the earliest to the latest. We should probably regard them as probably the most common and the most serious complication in small-pox. In many of the cases the lesions of the lung were so marked that they constituted a sufficient cause for death of the individual without the accompanying specific infection."[413]

Autopsy analysis cannot tell us of course what the outcome of an attack of smallpox would be on those who immediately survive the onslaught of the disease, although given the almost universal incidence of bronchitis and broncho-pneumonia among Councilman's cases and the emphasis that eighteenth century writers on smallpox placed on subsequent secondary mortality from lung diseases, it is difficult to resist the conclusion that indirect mortality from smallpox may well have been as high as Lettsom and others claimed. All these writers emphasized consumption as a secondary outcome of smallpox, and this is compatible with what is now known about the triggering of latent tuberculosis infection by other diseases. The tuberculosis bacillus can lie latent within human cells for very long periods—and then be released by a viral infection such as smallpox, which disrupts the structure of the cell.[414] Although this clearly is a topic which requires further specialized work before any firm conclusion can be reached, it does suggest that Lettsom and his contemporaries may have been right about the scale of secondary mortality from smallpox.

That smallpox is capable of producing serious long-term complications is illustrated by what we now know of its effect on the epididymis in males. Councilman and many other workers found much evidence of focal lesions in the testes and the epididymis through post-mortem analysis; of thirty cases studied in Councilman's sample, thirteen were found to have testicular lesions.[415] The most detailed work on this subject was carried out by Chiari, and Councilman summarized his findings on testicular lesions as follows:

"He found the lesions in fifteen cases of children, and in a further examination of sixty-three cases, mostly of adults, lesions were found in forty-five. The lesions showed a perfect agreement in their stage of development with the skin lesions . . . Chiari regards the affection as due to the direct action of the small-pox virus carried to the tissue by the blood. He thinks that in the testicle the conditions for action of the virus may be just as favourable as in the skin. The lesions show in their histological details similarity to the skin pocks."[416]

The similarity of skin lesions with those found in the testes was confirmed by Bras as recently as 1952; he found that

"The testicular lesions correlate with those of the skin; as a rule they occur after the onset of the vesicular stage and they can still be present when the skin lesions have healed."[417]

Although the persistence of these lesions in the testes was generally recognized, the possibility of them leading to male infertility tended to be discounted, until a very recently completed study revealed a high correlation between the presence of lesions in the epididymis and infertility.

A. M. Phadke and his colleagues published in 1973 their findings on research involving 8,000 patients who had registered at the Bombay Family Welfare Bureau during the previous nineteen years for treatment of infertility. I will summarize the conclusions of the study by quoting from it at some length:

"In 895 cases there was history and evidence of prior smallpox infection. These cases (designated the smallpox series) were analyzed according to the sperm counts and according to the lesions observed in the testicular biopsies. For the control series, another group of 895 serially registered infertile patients, who had not had smallpox, was analyzed in an identical way . . . the incidence of azoospermia [absence of viable sperms in the semen] was 42.57% in the smallpox series and only 17.87% in the control series. Likewise, the incidence of normospermia [normal amount of viable sperm in the semen] was only 30.17% in the smallpox series and as much as 52.52% in the control series . . . In clinical practice, the association of a history of smallpox infection with the occurrence of obstructive azoospermia is of proverbial frequency. The present study bears out the frequent clinical impression that the incidence of obstructive azoospermia is remarkably high in patients who have had the smallpox. Four of five such cases [in the azoospermia category] have obstructive lesions. The site of obstruction is usually at the lower end of the epididymis, and the testes miraculously seem to escape the brunt of the disease . . . In India, at least, obstructive azoospermia produced by smallpox infection in childhood frequently occurs . . . Smallpox infection is the most important and most frequently encountered single etiologic factor in India which produces obstructive azoospermia in man."[418]

I will discuss the demographic implications of these findings in the next chapter—we will see that there is some evidence for a correlation between changing smallpox mortality and changes in fertility—for the present, it is sufficient to note that smallpox is capable of inflicting life-long damage to vulnerable parts of the body, in ways not known about until very recently. It is probable that we shall never know with any exactness the full impact of the disease on overall mortality, given uncertainty about secondary causes of death such as broncho-pneumonia and the lack of research of the kind carried out by Phadke *et al* on male infertility.

One area on which there is very precise information on smallpox and its effects on mortality relates to pregnant women; it was recognized from a very early date—from at least the beginning of the eighteenth century—that pregnant women were highly vulnerable to the disease.[419] More recently, Rao and colleagues compared the outcome of smallpox in 94 pregnant women with that for a group of 348 matched non-pregnant cases in the Infectious Diseases Hospital at Madras; the overall fatality rate in the pregnant women was three times as high as that among the non-pregnant women, and in the twelve unvaccinated cases amongst the pregnant women, nine—75 per cent—died, compared to seventeen of the sixty-six (25.7 per cent) non-pregnant

women.[420] This scale of mortality among pregnant women who
caught smallpox is what might be expected from the historical
literature, and it is clear that this demographically critical group
was periodically decimated in country areas where the age-
incidence of the disease would make pregnant women vulnerable.
Rao *et al* speculate that this vulnerability may be due to the high
level of circulating cortieosteroid in the blood of pregnant women,
inhibiting the formation of antibodies; there is a fragment of
historical evidence that women were also more vulnerable to
smallpox during menstruation,[421] but the bearing that this has
on Rao's explanation of the vulnerability of pregnant women
is unclear.

In addition to the problem of the dark area of unknown
mortality due to the indirect effects of smallpox mortality (such
as broncho-pneumonia and infantile convulsions due to fulminating smallpox), there is the difficulty that we cannot assume that
smallpox was always registered even where it was known to be
the primary cause of death. Haygarth pointed out from his experience in Chester "that shopkeepers of almost all denominations, not only neglect every rule of prevention, but, lest their
trade should suffer, conceal, as much as possible, every instance
of the natural smallpox, which occurs in their families."[422]
Although it would have been difficult for such shopkeepers to
conceal death from smallpox in their families, they may have on
occasions been able to bribe the "searchers" who in places like
London were responsible for ascertaining the cause of death and
were described in 1783 as "women advanced in years and indigent
in circumstances."[423] Such a system of registration does not inspire
the greatest confidence in statistics derived from returns made
by the searchers. Many tradesmen in market towns may have
suppressed information about smallpox in their families and
certainly the townspeople as a whole were very anxious to avoid
advertising the presence of smallpox in their own town so as to
avoid frightening country people from the surrounding area—
there are many examples of markets being ruined for more than
a year because of the presence of smallpox. According to the local
historian of Dartford in Kent, in 1741 "the country people became
so alarmed that the market was nearly deserted, and did not
recover for some years."[424] Many of these market towns attempted
to isolate smallpox cases in the local Pest House, and according
to Dimsdale "due care is taken to bury the dead [from smallpox]
privately."[425] Not all these private burials at the Pest House were
registered in the parish register. When Mr Thomas Chubbs wrote
to Jurin on the 10th August 1723 to give his account of smallpox
in the town of Sarum, he stated that in addition to the 192 registered of dying from smallpox, "there have some died of that
Distemper, wch have been carried out of town to be buried, of
which I can recollect . . . 9, Tho' probably there may have been

more."[426] In this case, the proportion of private burials at the pest house does not appear to have been very large, but it is clear that there were occasions when such unregistered burials could be very large indeed; for example, the Maidstone parish register mentioned, but did not list by name, 102 children dying from smallpox in Maidstone in 1760 and "buried out of town."[427] As far as I am aware, no scholarly study has ever been carried out on the history of pest houses, and references to private burials are hard to come by, although they do occasionally occur in local histories; for example, at Hitchin in Hertfordshire: "1751. Paid John Person for a board to lay the dead on at the Folly, 1/6"— the Folly being the local Pest House.[428] If private burials of small-pox victims were as common as Dimsdale suggested, it could constitute a serious problem when trying to analyse smallpox mortality through parish registers. It is particularly unfortunate that where most statistical information on smallpox mortality is available—large towns and market towns—the registration of smallpox deaths is likely to have been most faulty. The inadequacy of registration was generally much greater in the large towns, for reasons which have been discussed, but it is again unfortunate that systematic statistics of smallpox mortality can only be compiled for large towns where bills of mortality were kept. Some parish registers of market towns do record death from smallpox, but it is not certain whether all smallpox deaths were recorded or whether some deaths were not registered through the casual nature of the registration procedure. Smallpox mortality and its change over time as depicted by statistics derived from bills of mortality and parish registers will be discussed later in the book.

CHAPTER 8
Smallpox Mortality Before the Introduction of Inoculation

One of the most reliable methods of estimating smallpox mortality throughout the eighteenth century is to multiply the proportion of the population suffering from the disease by its case-fatality rate, so that if 200 out of a population of 400 catch smallpox and 20 out of every 100 catching smallpox die from the disease, ten per cent of the population would have died from smallpox at that particular point of time. In general terms, in order to estimate the scale of smallpox mortality for the country as a whole it is necessary to estimate the proportion of the total population which caught the disease and then multiply by the estimated case-fatality rate for the whole country. This will be done in very general terms in the following discussion, starting with the attempt to estimate the proportion of the total population affected by smallpox.

Contemporaries during the eighteenth century were unanimous that smallpox was a disease that nearly everybody caught sooner or later, "almost every person must have it once."[429] D'Escheruy summed up contemporary opinion on the prevalence of smallpox:

". . . this distemper spares neither Age nor Sex; Rich and Poor are equally exposed to its Influence. What is the most unaccountable, and so wide from all other Fever, is, that the Difference of Constitution is no preservative against its Attack; inasmuch, that very few escape it, at one time or other . . ."[430]

D'Escheruy wrote this account in 1761 which is after the introduction of inoculation, but there is a great deal of evidence that smallpox was virtually a universal disease at a much earlier period. Smallpox appears to have been present in Europe at least since 581 A.D. when Gregory of Tours gave a very detailed description of the disease.[431] It was mentioned sporadically from then on until the late sixteenth century, when statistical evidence is available as to its prevalence. Between 1574 and 1598 the parish register of Allhallows, London Wall, contains information on the cause and age of death and during this twenty-five year period twelve people were listed as having died from smallpox. Ten of these twelve died under the age of seven years, the other two dying at the age of 12 and 30, the latter being a servant who had probably been recruited from the countryside.[432] This age distribution of those dying from smallpox suggests that the disease was sufficiently endemic in London to be a young child's disease. This is of course generally the case, i.e. where the disease returns every few years or so it will be almost exclusively a young child's disease as children are inevitably exposed to it within the first few years of life, and it being extremely rare for smallpox to attack the same person twice (the antibodies produced by the first attack usually protect for life), very few older people will be affected by it in this kind of epidemiological situation. It appears that smallpox was more or less endemic in most large towns by the early seventeenth century for it was a young child's disease in these places. According to the Kirk Session records of Aberdeen in 1610 "there was at this time a great visitation of the young children with the plague of the pocks"[433] and at Chester there was a note in the parish register in the year 1636 that "for this two or three yeares divers children dyed of small-pox in Chester."[434] From statistics of smallpox mortality during the eighteenth century it is clear that the disease was a very young child's disease in the large towns. Out of a total of 489 deaths from smallpox in Manchester during the period 1768-74, only 30 of them occurred above the age of five, the majority (366) taking place amongst children under the age of two.[435] During an earlier part of the eighteenth century, there are statistics on age and smallpox mortality for Kilmarnock, Scotland, during the period of 1728-62: the mean age at death from smallpox was 2.62 years and of a total of 613 smallpox deaths, 563 occurred under the age of five.[436].

It has sometimes been assumed that smallpox was a child's disease in all parts of Britain by the early part of the eighteenth century. We have previously discussed Monro's statement that smallpox was mainly a child's disease in Scotland and attempted to explain why this was the case, in terms of the Scottish peasantry's custom of visiting each other's family when a member was sick with smallpox. The English seem to have been much more careful when the disease was present in the vicinity and there is much evidence of the extreme lengths to which some people would go to avoid catching it; for example, a member of the Purefoy family who wrote to the Postmaster at Cheltenham in 1742:

"I having occasion to drink your waters at Cheltenham am oblidged to write to you, the Postmaster, to let me know if the small pox be at Cheltenham, if not I shall be there soon after I have your answer . . ."[437]

There is evidence of brothers refusing to attend the funerals of sisters because they had died of smallpox and brothers refusing to visit brothers because they had fallen sick of the disease.[438] We have seen how anxious the authorities of market towns were to deny rumours that smallpox was in the town because such rumours would ruin trade. The fear of smallpox not only led to the avoidance of places where the disease was present but also a fairly rigorous policy of isolation. Given the nature of smallpox, this is not at all surprising; what is more puzzling, is that the Scots do not appear to have shown the same fear of the disease— at least if Monro's account is to be accepted—and there is reason to believe that the Swedes had a very similar attitude. Sweden was one of the few countries in the eighteenth century with national statistics on smallpox, and it is therefore important to see what we can learn from them about the universality of the disease. The following is the age incidence of the yearly average number of smallpox deaths in the period 1774-1798:

Yearly Average Number of Smallpox Deaths at Various Ages, Sweden, 1774-1798[439]

Age Group (Years)	Under 1 Year	1-3	3-5	5-10	Above 10	All Ages
Average Smallpox Deaths	1137	1223	870	585	306	4131
%'s	27.5	29.6	21.1	14.2	7.4	99.8

Only 7.4 per cent of smallpox deaths were over the age of ten, and the vast majority—78.2 per cent—were under five. What is very surprising about these figures is that Sweden was a very rural country at this time, with much of its population living under very isolated conditions. It is possible that some of the older members of the population had been inoculated previous to the compilation of the statistics, although the little evidence that is available does not support this.[440] The figures as they stand indicate that smallpox was a universal disease— everyone more or less catching the disease as a young child. Although we do not have similar national figures for Britain, the evidence we do have strongly suggests that smallpox was not exclusively a disease of young children in the first half of the eighteenth century. In Sweden epidemics seemed to have occurred every five years or so; in many parts of England, epidemics appeared at very much longer intervals, as is indicated in the following Table summarizing evidence from a number of local sources.

Periodicity of Smallpox Epidemics in Provincial England

Place	Date of Epidemics				
Skipton-in-Craven, Yorks[441]	1716-17	1723	1726-27	1732	1736
Maidstone, Kent[442]	1734	1741	1745	1753	1760
Taunton, Somerset[443]	1658	1670	1677	1684	
Sherbourne, Dorset[444]	1634	1642-43	1649-50	1657-58	1667
Godalming, Surrey[445]	1672	1686	1701	1710-11	1723-24

The periodicity of epidemics in these places varied from a minimum of about every five years in Skipton-in-Craven to a maximum of about every 12½ years in Godalming, Surrey, with the other places lying somewhere in between. The factors determining the periodicity of epidemics were the total size of the population of the place and its degree of geographical isolation from the rest of the country. A small relatively isolated village is likely to have had epidemics only infrequently, and when such epidemics did occur they would affect the majority of the population, adults as well as children, as many children would grow to adulthood without being attacked by the disease. An example of this is to be found at Aynho, Northants, which was a village with a population of about 350 in 1723-24 when the epidemic occurred to which the Table below refers:[446]

Ages (Years)	0-10	10-20	20-30	30-40	40-50	50-60	60
Smallpox Cases	28	47	25	12	10	4	6

Over forty per cent of all smallpox attacks in this epidemic occurred amongst adults of 20 years and above; this age distribution can only occur when epidemics return relatively infrequently. The exact periodicity of epidemics in Aynho is unknown, but it must have been very similar to that in Godalming, Surrey, where 81 of the total of 151 people who died from smallpox in the period 1701-24 were children, i.e. epidemics returning about every twelve or thirteen years. Not all the population in Aynho were attacked during the 1723-24 epidemic but this was probably because many of them had caught the disease in previous epidemics. There is some statistical information as to the proportion of the population which escaped from an attack of smallpox and had not had the disease.

Smallpox Census of Ware, Herts., in 1722[447]

Number of Families	Number of People	"Had Ye Smallpox Before"	"Had Ye Smallpox This Time"	"To Have Smallpox"	Died of Smallpox
564	2515	1601	612	302	72

It is important to note that Mr Anthony Fage, a surgeon at Ware who compiled these statistics in order to answer the enquiry sent out by Jurin about smallpox mortality, included the 302 people who escaped smallpox and had not had it previously under the heading *"To Have Smallpox."* He assumed that they would be bound to catch the disease sooner or later, not an unreasonable assumption in the light of the statistics returned: a total of 684 people caught the disease in 1722, 1601 had caught it previously, leaving only 302 who had not been attacked by the disease. It is known that very few people are immune from attack by small-pox, and if frequently exposed to the disease (as all people must have been in Ware) virtually all will catch it. Another example of a similar smallpox census is that carried out by Frewen, a surgeon, after the smallpox epidemic in Hastings during 1730-32:

Smallpox Census of Hastings, Sussex 1730-32[48]

Recovered from Smallpox (including four that were inoculated)	Died of it	Escaped it	Died of other diseases since the smallpox raged there	Total Population
608	97	206	50	1636

During this epidemic in 1730-32 over 700 people caught smallpox (of which 97 died) and at least 725 had caught the disease previously—only 206 escaped it. The number catching the disease was nearly half the total population, which suggests that epidemics were relatively infrequent in the town, but it is clear that most of the population were prone to smallpox sooner or later.

Although the conclusion that smallpox was a universal disease before the introduction of inoculation would seem obvious from the evidence so far considered, there is some evidence to the contrary. The parish register of Riseley, Beds., lists all the causes of deaths between 1690 and 1742 and there appears to have been no epidemic of smallpox at all during this period—there were one or two smallpox deaths every five years or so, in all a total of 27 deaths from smallpox during the whole period. This might be partly due to the fact that no cause of death was given for "infants" who constituted over a fifth of the total deaths—many of these "infants" might have died from small-pox; alternatively many of the smallpox victims might have been buried privately at the local pest house. It is possible that either the spread of smallpox was prevented by successful isolation of those sick or that the case-fatality rate was particularly low in this parish—the latter seems unlikely, as we shall see in subsequent discussion. It is also difficult to see how smallpox cases could have been so successfully isolated over such a long period of time, particularly in the light of the pattern of smallpox mortality summarized in the following table:

Smallpox Deaths in Riseley, Beds., 1690-1742[49]

Date	1690	1701	1702	1703	1710	1714	1715
Smallpox Deaths	4	1	5	2	1	1	3

Date	1716	1720	1722	1724	1725	1732	1740
Smallpox Deaths	2	1	2	1	2	2	1

One would have expected the presence of smallpox in the parish during the periods 1701-03 and 1714-16 to have led to at least one significant epidemic. Riseley is estimated to have had a population of 425 in 1671 and an enumerated population of 576 in 1801.[450] Such a village could normally expect an epidemic every ten years or so, if other statistical evidence is anything to go by. Even in so isolated a parish as the peninsular Isle of Purbeck in Dorset—described by the local incumbent in 1803 as "my insulated parish and neighbourhood"—appears to have had smallpox epidemics about every twenty years, although during the previous forty years to which the incumbent was writing, the parish had been affected by smallpox, "once by infection, and once by inoculation."[451]

There are very good theoretical grounds for believing however that if epidemics did not occur at all during a very prolonged period—say the fifty-two year period 1690-1742 considered in Riseley—the population would become highly genetically vulnerable to a disease like smallpox, leading to eventual massive mortality. Populations which are not affected by fairly frequent epidemics which kill off a proportion of their members, become genetically vulnerable to future attacks through the survival of people with low natural resistance to the disease. Frequent epidemics kill off the biologically vulnerable, who are therefore unable to pass on their genes to future generations; there is therefore a process of natural selection at work, with those highly vulnerable disappearing from the population. This theoretical expectation is more than borne out by the historical literature. Communities which were very geographically isolated suffered from very infrequent epidemics, which when they did arrive, were very fatal. An example of this occurred in Greenland in the first half of the eighteenth century:

"Smallpox was first brought to Greenland, in the year 1734, by a vessel from Denmark. Nearly two-thirds of the whole population of that country (which at that time was from 6000 to 7000) were swept away by this disease. Of 200 families living within a circle of from two to three miles from the Danish settlement into which the smallpox was brought, not 30 remained alive."[452]

The only similar case which is known to have occurred in Britain is that when

"in 1720, the disease was so fatal as to be distinguished by the name of the mortal pox. On this occasion tradition tells us, in the remote Island of Foula, probably inhabited by about two hundred people, it left only four to six to bury the dead."[453]

The Island of Foula is one of the Shetland Islands and is naturally isolated from the Scottish mainland, being eighteen miles from the nearest land. There are no examples of other spectacular fatalities on this scale to be found in the British literature, although Holwell in his treatise on Indian inoculation noted a similar phenomena for the isolated island of St Helena (presumably the same remote Atlantic island that Napoleon was exiled to):

"It is singularly worth remarking that there hardly ever was an instance of a native of the Island of St Helena, man or woman, that was seized with this distemper in the natural way (when resident in Bengall) who escaped with life; although it is a known fact the disease never yet got footing upon that Island."[454]

The massive fatality of smallpox amongst the American Indians is also well-known,[455] and the same process of genetic vulnerability was presumably at work in all these instances.

Thus the absence of highly fatal epidemics in Britain except for that found in Foula indicates that the population was periodically affected by the disease, either in endemic forms in the large towns or in epidemics in the countryside. Practically everybody sooner or later appears to have been infected by the disease, and this is reflected in the contemporary literature of the period. As early as the beginning of the seventeenth century Ben Jonson wrote in his "Epigram to the Small Pox"—"Envious and foule Disease, could there not be One beautie in an Age, and free from thee?"[456] During a later part of the century in 1674 Mr Z. Isham, a Northamptonshire country gentleman, wrote to his brother Sir J. Isham in connection with a smallpox epidemic in the neighbourhood:

"I have no reason on my own particular to be very secure, having never yet had that almost Universall Disease."[457]

This type of statement indicates in general terms that smallpox was widely prevalent even in the countryside. There is a great deal of evidence that most parishes expected smallpox to die out during an epidemic only after it had attacked most of the population at risk. According to a letter sent in 1723 to Jurin in connection with his enquiry into smallpox mortality, "about ten or twelve years ago the small pox went thro' their parish (Bradpole near Bridport) and few escaped it, at that time seven score were sick."[458] Similarly, one of the Purefoy family wrote in a letter in 1736 that "our town of Buckingham is grievously visited with the small pox, the last I hear of it, it was in three score houses, so forasmuch as it is so universall hope it will be soon over."[459] It is of course possible that some parishes managed to avoid epidemics altogether by effectively isolating those sick from smallpox. Most parish registers which give information about the disease indicate that epidemics sooner or later occurred; Thomas Short, who made a very thorough contemporary study of diseases, concluded that in the case of smallpox, "the Disease keeps certain Periods of Return; as once in three or four years in large Towns, or six or seven years in wild, moorish country Places . . ."[460] He seems to have been referring to epidemics, with which he was mainly concerned; perhaps his conclusion is an approximate summary of what was happening in most parts of the country, although as we have seen epidemics did occur in places like Godalming at much greater intervals of time. Short did make it clear that smallpox was endemic in the country as a whole and stated that "there is no general Constitution of Weather wherein the Smallpox are not epidemic somewhere . . . [and sometimes] we shall find them in one Village, Parish, Town, or Corner of a County, and no where else in the Kingdom."[461] I have previously pointed out that smallpox appears to have been present in London every week during the seventeenth and eighteenth centuries (according to the Bills of Mortality) and therefore London formed a kind of smallpox reservoir from which the disease was continually exported to the country at large.

The evidence that Jurin collected as secretary of the Royal Society on the comparative mortality of smallpox and inoculation, provided quite a bit of incidental information on the extent of the natural form of the diseases. Jurin himself assumed in his calculations that "there are great Numbers, that never have the Small Pox",[462] but unfortunately he displayed only a limited grasp of the epidemiological problems confronting him. One of his correspondents, Mr Towgood of Shepton Mallet in Somerset, wrote arguing that he could statistically demonstrate the fallacy of the argument that people could escape natural smallpox even in a rural area of the kind in which he was living in. He wrote to Jurin about

> "the Result of an Attempt I have been upon, but thro' hurry of business have not been able to finish. Tis a Computation of what proportion persons above 25 years old that never had the Small Pox bear to the rest of Mankind that have had them. For this end I have fixed on a middle Street of this Town, which is a considerable Place of Trade; and a Village on the skirt of the Town; and on a large Scattered Parish in the Country where there are Scarce two Houses contiguous. I imagine a Calculation made out of these 3 . . . would . . . give no Small Evidence on the Side of Inoculation in Answer to that Clamour so common among us in these parts, that the Inoculated in a great measure run a needless hazard, for they might never have the distemper in the natural way."[463]

Although Towgood had obviously collected some information on the problem—presumably an initial house-to-house enquiry—he had not been able to finish his calculations because of pressure of work in his medical practice. Unfortunately, Jurin dissuaded

him from completing his research on the spurious grounds that
the risk of dying from natural smallpox was already known from
calculations based on the London Bills of Mortality! Smallpox
was of course an endemic childhood disease in London, most
people catching it by the age of seven; in Somerset it would have
been an epidemic disease—in Taunton as we have seen it returned every six or seven years or so at the end of the seventeenth century—and the age incidence would have been much
higher.

Jurin did however inadvertently collect some national statistics
which throw some further light on this problem; not only did he
collect information on the number of people inoculated, but also
their ages. Although we cannot assume that these inoculated
cases were representative of the population at risk to smallpox—
they were undoubtedly disproportionately selected from the
wealthier social classes, and probably also from the towns—
they do give some idea of the age structure of the vulnerable
population. The following is an age breakdown of the 477 people
inoculated by 1724:[164]

Age	Number Inoculated	Percentage (of Total)
Under One Year	11	2.3%
One Year to Two	15	3.1%
Two to Three	31	6.5%
Three to Four	41	8.6%
Four to Five	33	6.9%
Five to Ten	143	30.0%
Ten to Fifteen	82	17.2%
Fifteen to Twenty	56	11.7%
Twenty to Fifty-Two	62	13.0%
Age Unknown	3	0.6%

There were only about thirteen per cent inoculated above the
age of twenty, and none above the age of fifty-two; these figures
as they stand clearly indicate that most people had caught the
disease by the age of twenty, most of those at risk being under
that age. Although the figures on which this conclusion is based
are not necessarily representative of all social and geographically
located groups, they are at least national data, and are probably
the best source of information for estimating the national age-
incidence of smallpox, and therefore indirectly its degree of
universality in the population.

I have assumed in the discussion to date that everyone
in the population is biologically vulnerable to smallpox if sufficiently exposed to the disease—thus the epidemiological assumption that age incidence will reveal the extent of the disease in the
population (if everyone is biologically vulnerable and all who die

are children, everyone must have caught the disease as children—otherwise, there would be people dying at a later age after childhood). There is good evidence however that a small minority is biologically totally immune to the disease, and it may have been this minority that Jurin and others had in mind when referring to some people escaping the illness altogether. Gatti summarized in 1767 the contemporary consensus of opinion, which would probably now be accepted as valid:

"It is certain, there are some who never have it [smallpox]; whole families are free from it for many generations; and it has been observed, that upon a hundred persons dying of old age, five or six had escaped it, though equally exposed to their contemporaries. Inoculators have met with much the same proportion of fruitless attempts."[465]

Gatti could come to such a precise conclusion because of his great knowledge of the history of inoculation, as well as his observation of smallpox over nearly a fifty year period.

Most contemporaries agreed that smallpox was a universal disease which sooner or later more-or-less affected everyone. Sloane argued in 1735 in favour of inoculation on the grounds that "since it is reckoned, that scarce one in a thousand misses having it some time in their life, the sooner it is given them the better."[466] Its universality was sufficiently great to give rise to the theory of humoral pathology—that it was an innate contagion which had to be discharged and expressed through the blood—and Hillary summarized this view in 1740:

"Nor have we any Account of the Small Pox or Measles, till about the Year 640; tho' they are now become so universal Disease as any we know of . . . This Disease [smallpox] being so universal, it induced those who first wrote upon it, to believe that Infants before their Births contracted a seminal Contagion, a **sanguine mestruoso matris (m)** . . . This Opinion was constantly received and believed, till the Discovery of the Circulation of the Blood . . . exploded this ill-grounded **Arabian** hypothesis . . ."[467]

Hillary was premature in believing "this ill-grounded **Arabian** Hypothesis" to have been completely exploded, for as late as 1767 Bromfield was arguing "from the universality of this disease [smallpox] amongst mankind in most places, it seems, as if nature had some salutary end for the constitution, to be answered by this depuration that the blood undergoes at such time."[468] Such views now seem absurd to us, but the combination of the inevitability of catching the disease with such a high risk of fatality made a marked impression on many of the people who wrote on the subject; for example, in 1752 Thompson concluded

"There is no disease to which mankind is unhappily subject, so fatal in its effects, so universal in its influence, which so deeply affects the minds of all people . . ."[469]

The belief in the inevitability of smallpox continued to be held by medical writers until the end of the eighteenth century. In 1779 Benjamin Pugh, a surgeon, wrote from Baddow near Chelmsford in Essex that

"There is, I believe, scarcely an instance to be produced, in town or village, where any escaped the infection before inoculation was in use; and I have known many who have escaped so long, that they have been persuaded they never should have the small-pox, and yet have died of the confluent kind in extreme old age."[470]

Similarly, another surgeon William Black wrote in 1781:

". . . but even in country villages, I imagine that very few are grown up to the age of twenty, who either have not had the Small-Pox, or have not been several times exposed within the sphere of variolous effluvia."[471]

Haygarth in 1793 butressed the conclusion about the inevitability of smallpox with some statistics on smallpox among the Cheshire and Lancashire militia:

"In this neighbourhood [of Chester], neither in town nor country, no considerable number, who are capable of receiving the distemper, escape till they are men and women. To establish the truth of this remark, in 1781, I learned from Mr Edwards, surgeon in the Cheshire militia, that all the regiment had been infected except **thirty** in **six hundred, or one** in **twenty**, the proportion naturally exempted from it through life. When the Lancashire militia was in Chester, I made the same inquiry of Mr Drinkwater, their surgeon. He informed me that nearly the same proportion of them had passed through the smallpox."[472]

Only a very small minority of the militia appeared to have been inoculated, for Haygarth was informed in 1782 that only six of 466 of them had been previously inoculated;[473] given that most of these men would have caught smallpox in the pre-Suttonian era as children, this confirms our earlier conclusion about the relatively insignificant practice of inoculation in the earlier period (although many of these men may have come from Chester and other towns where inoculation was less practised anyway). The universality of smallpox among these men cannot be attributed to secondary contagion from inoculation, as it was much too rare to be a major source of infection.

The mortality from a disease is of course a function of both its incidence in a population, and its case-fatality rate. Four main factors can be identified as influencing case-fatality: (1) the genetic vulnerability of the population depending upon the periodicity of epidemics as already discussed; (2) the age structure of the population, some age groups having higher case-fatality rates than others; (3) the virulence of the particular smallpox virus leading to the outbreak in question; (4) the hygienic conditions of the population and the presence or absence of other diseases and biological states. I have already indicated that there is little evidence for high genetic vulnerability to smallpox in Britain during the eighteenth century; however, there does seem to have been examples of high mortality, which may have been based on epidemiologically linked processes of natural selection. For example, Lettsom noted that

"in some countries, and even some counties of England, the infection does not appear for the space of some years; but when it does appear, it is more fatal; owing probably to this, that in great towns the infection being always prevalent, it is caught without the accumulated changes of air peculiarly favourable to epidemics; whereas when it comes at stated periods, its malignity seems to be augmented by some unknown but deleterious state of the atmosphere."[474]

Lettsom was of course unaware of the possibility of any kind of explanation in terms of natural selection, but the observations he made would be consistent with people in isolated country areas suffering from more fatal smallpox on account of greater genetic vulnerability. There are a number of instances of high rural mortality which might be illustrations of this point; Eversley has noted the very fatal epidemic of smallpox which occurred in the eleven villages and one town in the area of Bromsgrove, Worcs., during the period 1725-29[475] It wiped out more than a fifth of the population of Hanbury during 1725, which according to Eversley is a conservative estimate. Only about a third of the smallpox deaths were of children, which indicates that the majority of the population was attacked and thus suggests that the last epidemic had taken place many years previously. Another example of a spectacular smallpox epidemic during the eighteenth century is that which took place at Burford, Oxon., in 1758. Burford was a very small market town with a population of about 1200, located in a relatively isolated position within the Cotswolds.[476] In the parish register for the year of 1758 is a list of all the persons who died of smallpox in that year, which is summarized at the end by the simple statement that "190 persons died of the Small-Pox."[477] Even this is probably an under-enumeration as the total burials were as follows: 1754 - 28; 1755 - 41; 1756 - 39; 1757 - 43; 1758 - 240; 1759 - 41; 1760 - 33; 1761 - 27; 1762 - 34. This 1758 epidemic only lasted about four months; 185 of the 190 recorded smallpox deaths occurred between 10th April and 28th July, during which time there was a total of 199 deaths. It is safe to assume that there were at least 200 deaths from smallpox, and it is known that over a half of the total occurred amongst children, suggesting that the case-fatality rate was very high, *i.e.* about 200 people died from smallpox amongst a population of about 1200, not all of whom were attacked by the disease (if all the population had been attacked, a higher proportion of deaths would have occurred amongst adults). Spectacular epidemics of the kind at Hanbury and Burford were sufficiently common for McKenzie to write in 1760 "that when small-pox is epidemic, entire villages are depopulated, markets ruined, and the face of distress spread over the whole country."[478]

The weight of the evidence is however against the genetic vulnerability hypothesis; not only does previously considered evidence suggest that smallpox was a more-or-less universal disease affecting nearly all the population, even in rural areas, but even some of the examples quoted of spectacular epidemics lead to the same conclusion. Over half the people dying from smallpox in Burford were children, suggesting fairly regular and frequent epidemics of the kind that would kill off the genetically vulnerable. Also, there is some evidence to suggest that smallpox mortality was sometimes **lower** in rural areas than in urban ones. For example, an anonymous correspondent of Jurin's wrote to him on the 23rd February 1723, making the following point:

". . . a Friend of mine that lives at Bradpole near Bridport [Dorset] informs me, That about ten or twelve years ago the small Pox went thro their parish and few escaped it, at that time seven score were sick whereof no more than six or seven dyed. He saith twas at Lother a Neighbouring parish about the same time, and the Number of them that dyded there was as small in proportion to the Number of the Sick as at Bradpole: the Number of them that dye of the Small pox in Country Parishes is in Proportion to the Sick much less than in populous Towns and Cityes."[479]

On the other hand, another of Jurin's correspondents pointed out at about the same time that about one in five died from smallpox in the town of Portsmouth and its neighbouring area, whereas "Havant a Village seven miles hence lost even more."[480] Nettleton had claimed that "the Proportion of those that die is much the same" in the town and country,[481] but as Haygarth had pointed out at the end of the eighteenth century, fatality rates were greatly influenced by the age incidence of the disease and this usually varied between the town and countryside.[482] It is partly possible to examine this question by comparing the small number of non-industrial rural villages in Jurin's sample of communities in the smallpox censuses of the 1720's, with the remaining sample of towns and industrial villages. There were seven non-industrial villages—Hatherfield, Havant, Dedham, Aynho, Cobham, Kempsey and Uxbridge—and of 1234 cases of smallpox, 298 died, a case-fatality of 24.1 per cent; this compares with 11,958 cases and 1869 deaths—a case-fatality rate of 15.6 per cent—in the remaining 25 towns and industrial villages in the sample.[483] Although this difference is a fairly significant one, it is of a scale that is more likely to be explained by variations in age incidence, than the relatively dramatic factors involved in genetic selectivity.

Virtually the only evidence of the effect of age-incidence on mortality in the eighteenth century came from data sent to Jurin on the smallpox epidemic at the small village of Aynho in Northamptonshire in 1723-24. The following is a summary of that evidence.

Smallpox Mortality at Aynho, Northants, 1723-24[484]

Age (Years)	Cases	Deaths	Percentage Fatality
0-10	28	4	14.3
10-20	47	4	8.5
20-30	25	6	24.0
30-40	12	3	25.0
40+	20	8	40.0

Although some of these figures are based on very small numbers, the pattern to emerge is very similar to that found in larger nineteenth century surveys. For example, the following is a summary of data available for a very large series of cases reported in Berlin, Germany for the years 1865-74:

Smallpox Mortality Amongst the Unvaccinated at Berlin, 1865-74[485]

Age (Years)	Cases	Deaths	Percentage Fatality
0-10	5270	2124	40
10-20	218	25	12
20-30	316	57	18
30-40	196	52	27
40+	213	83	39

Both the Aynho and Berlin figures reveal a U-shaped distribution, although the U is much more even in Berlin than in Aynho; minimum mortality was found in both surveys to be amongst the 10-20 year age group, and the maximum mortality—found at the extremes of the age spectrum—was of the order of four times as

great. The Aynho figures indicate that the under ten age group
had a relatively low fatality rate and this is almost certainly a
function of the smallness of the numbers involved; all the nineteenth century surveys showed peaks of mortality at both the
younger and older age ranges, and this was most vividly illustrated
by the figures of smallpox mortality at Homerton Smallpox Hospital (London), which because of the number of cases were broken
down into very detailed age categories.

*Smallpox Mortality Amongst the Unvaccinated at Homerton
Smallpox Hospital, 1870-83*[486]

Age (Years)	Cases	Deaths	Percentage Fatality
Under One	155	98	63.2
1- 2	121	83	68.5
2- 3	115	77	61.6
3- 4	129	65	46.7
4- 5	147	60	41.3
5-10	510	180	35.2
10-15	317	74	23.3
15-20	204	86	42.3
20-25	174	83	47.7
25-30	105	56	53.3
30-35	53	22	41.5
35-40	50	20	40.0
40+	79	34	43.0

In Homerton Hospital although the U-curve distribution is still
present, the peak mortality occurs in the very young age groups,
particularly under the age of three. Most of these surveys show
a significant minimum mortality among the 10-20 age group,
but in the Homerton figures it is more specifically the 10-15 age
group which is at the bottom of the U distribution. The scale of
differences is so significant—at Homerton of the order of three to
one—that we must clearly allow for age incidence when we are
discussing the overall problem of smallpox mortality and how
it changed over time.

All the evidence points to a gradual but highly significant
increase in the virulence and case-fatality rate of smallpox from
the late sixteenth through to the end of the nineteenth century
when it sharply began to decline. Before discussing this evidence,
we may summarize McVail's conclusions reached through a detailed examination of some of the sources:

"... natural smallpox gradually became throughout the
eighteenth century, and up to the epidemic of 1870-73, a
more virulent and fatal disease, its maximum fatality being
on a large basis of facts 45 per cent, and since then it has
irregularly, yet persistently, diminished in fatality until we

come to the epidemic of 1902-5 with unvaccinated rate of 19.3 per cent."[487]

Although this conclusion applies to the eighteenth and nineteenth centuries, the increase in the virulence of smallpox almost certainly started as late as the end of the sixteenth century. This was reflected in the increasing mortality from smallpox in London during the seventeenth century.

Percentage of All Deaths due to
Smallpox in London[488]

Period	Percentage
1574-98	1.6
1629-36	2.8
1650-60	4.8
1660-70	3.6
1670-80	7.1
1680-90	7.3
1690-1700	4.5
1700-10	5.3
1710-20	8.1
1720-30	8.2

Although these statistics of smallpox mortality in London are unreliable as indications of total mortality due to smallpox (for reasons already discussed), they do indicate the increase in the fatality of the disease during the period 1574-1730. As the statistics refer to the same type of environment where smallpox was throughout the whole period a disease of young children, it would appear that the increase in fatality was due to an increase in the virulence of the disease. There do seem to have been fluctuations in the virulence of smallpox during the period, with a first peak during 1670-90 and a second in 1710-30. The increase in virulence during the middle of the seventeenth century is reflected in contemporary comments; for example Dr Tobias Whitaker, who had been exiled with Charles II during the civil war, wrote in 1661 that smallpox

"was constantly and generally in the common place of **petit** and **puerile** and the cure of no moment . . . But from what present constitution of ague this childish disease hath received such pestilential tinctures I know not; yet I am sure that this disease, which for hundreds of yeares and before the practice of medicine was so exquisite, hath been as commonly cured as it hapned . . ."[489]

Other commentators writing in the 1660s noticed this increase in the fatality of smallpox,[490] but as late as 1689 Dr Walter Harris could write:

129

"Smallpox and measles in infants, being for the most part a
mild and tranquil effervesence of the blood, are wont to have
often no bad character, where neither the helping hand of
physicians are called, nor the unbounding skill of complacent
nurses is put in requisition."[491]

There was some decline in virulence during the period 1690-1710
according to the London statistics, followed by an increased virulence after the 1710s, which as we shall see later continued
throughout the eighteenth and nineteenth centuries. The increase
in virulence after the 1710s in London seems to have occurred
somewhat later in the country at large, as is illustrated by the
following figures:

*Deaths from Smallpox in Godalming, Surrey
and Skipton-in-Craven, Yorks.*[492]

Period	Godalming Deaths from Smallpox	Period	Skipton-in-Craven Deaths from Smallpox
1636	50	1716-22	13
1701	24	1723-29	51
1710-11	39	1730-36	54
1722-23	94		

These statistics only refer to two towns and as smallpox mortality is known to vary greatly from one epidemic to another
depending upon the particular virus causing the epidemic (as
will be discussed in a moment), we must be careful about the conclusions we reach from such evidence. However, all the available
evidence does point to a general increase in virulence from the
1720s onwards; for example, according to the Basingstoke parish
register which lists smallpox deaths, 50 people died during the
1714 epidemic, whereas 125 died from the same disease during
1741. The increase in virulence is also reflected in contemporary
comment; the compiler of the *Northampton Bills of Mortality*
noted in 1740 that "the Small-Pox has been very much in this
Town this Year, and more mortal by far than in any one Year
in the Memory of Man."[493] Similarly Deering noted in 1751 that
the smallpox epidemic of 1736 in Nottingham

"was a fatal Instance, for from the latter End of May to the
beginning of September, this Distemper [smallpox] swept
away a great Number of Souls (but mostly Children) and in
the single Month of May, there were buried in St Mary's
Church and Church-yard only, 104; in short, the Burials
exceeded that Year the Births by above 380, whereas otherwise there is **communibus annis** an increase of about 65; a

Mortality, the like I have not been able to discover in looking back into the Church Registers for above 30 years, and I much question whether there has been the like since the Plague, which visited this Town in 1667, and made a cruel Desolation in the higher part of Nottingham . . ."[494]

Creighton in his historical survey of smallpox epidemics in Britain emphasized the virulence of smallpox during the early 1720s:

"The years 1722 and 1723 . . . were one of the greater smallpox periods in England. In Short's abstracts of the parish registers those years stand out very prominently by reason of the excess of deaths over births in a large proportion of country parishes; and according to Wintringham's annals, it was not fever that made them fatal years, but smallpox, along with autumnal dysentries and diarrhoeas."[495]

Creighton was much too much influenced by the evidence immediately available to him, and as we have already seen smallpox was very fatal after the early 1720s in the Bromsgrove area, Nottingham, Northampton, Burford etc. Before considering the general evidence on the change of virulence during the eighteenth and nineteenth centuries, it is necessary to discuss in some detail the statistics of smallpox mortality compiled by Jurin and others during the 1720s, which provide the most accurate and general account of smallpox mortality before the introduction of popular inoculation.

Twenty-six of the thirty-two censuses were conducted in market towns: in no sense must they be taken as a comprehensive census of all the smallpox epidemics in the 1720s. They appear to have been epidemics which caught the attention of a few medical practitioners and others who were interested in reporting them for statistical purposes; Nettleton of Halifax was responsible for reporting twelve epidemics and thus the predominance of Yorkshire in 1722. The overall case-fatality rate derived from all the censuses was 16.5 per cent, *i.e.* of 13,192 people catching smallpox, 2167 (16.5 per cent) died. There was considerable variation in the case-fatality rate from one epidemic to another—the minimum was 9.1 per cent at Deal during 1725-26, the maximum at Uxbridge in 1727, 36.4 per cent. It was noted in connection with the smallpox census at Uxbridge, that "at Uxbridge and in the neighbourhood, the smallpox having been exceedingly fatal all thereabouts".[496] The variation in the fatality of smallpox was well recognized by contemporaries, "it is sometimes so very Mortal, and at other Times so very Mild and Favourable"[497] and "they are fatal in one Place, favourable in another and not known in a third".[498] This clearly means that statistics of mortality from any one place can be very misleading as an indication of general mortality in the country as a whole, al-

Censuses of Smallpox Epidemics in England, 1721-31[499]

Locality of the Epidemic	Date	Cases	Deaths	Per Cent Fatality
Halifax	1721-22	276	43	15.9
Rochdale	,,	177	38	21.4
Leeds	,,	792	189	23.8
Halifax	1722	565	87	15.4
Bradford	,,	129	36	27.9
Wakefield	,,	418	57	13.6
Ashton-under-Lyme	,,	279	56	20.0
Macclesfield	,,	302	37	12.2
Stockport	,,	287	73	25.4
Hatherfield	,,	180	20	11.1
Chichester	,,	994	168	16.9
Haverfordwest	,,	227	52	22.9
Barstand, Ripponden Scorby and part of Halifax parish 4 miles from town	,,	230	38	16.5
Bolton	1723	406	89	21.6
Ware	,,	612	72	11.7
Salisbury	,,	1244	165	13.2
Romsey, Hants.	,,	913	143	15.6
Havant	,,	264	61	23.1
Bedford	,,	786	147	18.4
Shaftesbury	1724	660	100	15.1
Dedham, near Colchester	,,	339	106	31.3
Plymouth	,,	188	32	17.2
Aynho, near Banbury	1723-24	133	25	18.8
Stratford-on-Avon	1724	562	89	15.8
Bolton-le-Moor	,,	341	64	18.8
Cobham	,,	105	20	19.0
Dover	1725-26	503	61	12.1
Deal	,,	362	33	9.1
Kempsey, near Worcester	1726	73	15	20.5
Uxbridge	1727	140	51	36.4
Hastings	1730-31	705	97	13.7
		13,192	2167	16.5

though the degree of variation in the case-fatality rate in the censuses of the 1720s is not that great, most epidemics having a case-fatality rate near the average (16.5 per cent). This average figure is probably unrepresentative of the country as a whole inasmuch as a disproportionate number of industrial market towns are included in the sample, and it appears that most cases of smallpox in these areas occurred amongst children. Of seventy-eight people inoculated by Nettleton in the Halifax area in 1723,

83 per cent of them were under the age of seven, with a median age of approximately four years.[500] Presumably therefore in these areas most people caught smallpox after the age of four at some time during their younger childhood. In a rural area like Aynho on the other hand, many people caught smallpox during their adulthood, with the result that the case-fatality rate of that village was slightly above average. We have seen that case-fatality in the seven non-industrialized villages in the smallpox census sample was 24.1 per cent, and this higher than average fatality rate was probably due to the greater population of adults affected in rural areas. It is therefore likely that the figures derived from the smallpox censuses understate the national case-fatality rate during the 1720s, as most of the population would have been living in small villages rather than towns and industrial areas.

The relevance of age to smallpox mortality was certainly recognized by contemporaries; for example, the Rev David Some writing in 1725 stated "that of young Children that have it, one in six or seven commonly die of it; and of grown Persons, at least one in three."[501] This fits quite well with what we know of the relationship between age and case-fatality rates, although there are marked variations within the childhood category which influence smallpox mortality. An illustration of this is found in the writings of Isaac Massey, one of the early opponents of inoculation; in 1723 he claimed that among the children of the Christ's Hospital school, "not One out of fifty have died these last twenty years of that Distemper [smallpox]"[502]—a figure which may well have been accurate, as all the children in the school were between the ages of eight and fifteen, the period of minimal case-fatality. These variations in fatality and mortality rates illustrate the danger of taking isolated examples as in any way representative; it is necessary always to take evidence from a number of different sources and places—such as the smallpox censuses of the 1720s—and place it in a general context of what is known about the influence of a variable like age.

The low fatality amongst the Christ's Hospital children may also have been partly a function of what appears from the London mortality figures to have been a dip in the virulence of the disease, at least for the period 1690-1710. The Rev Some claimed in 1725 "that of late Years, it [smallpox] has been more mortal than usual."[503] It is possible that some of this increase in mortality was due to a deterioration in hygiene—poor hygiene is thought to increase the fatality of smallpox[504]—but there is evidence that the case-fatality rate was rising independently of environmental conditions during the eighteenth century. The following summarizes changes in case-fatality rates in the second half of the eighteenth and first half of the nineteenth century in the London Smallpox Hospital, which as far as is known provided a fairly homogeneous environment during the whole period.

Case-Fatality Rate of Smallpox in London Smallpox Hospital[505]

Period	Number of Cases	Percentage that Died
1746-63	6456	25½
1776-1800	7017	32
1836-51	2654	38

The London Smallpox Hospital was moved from its original site to a new hospital at St Pancras at the end of the eighteenth century, and it is therefore unlikely that the increase in case-fatality was due to a deterioration in hygiene. It is also possible that there was a change in the age distribution of patients admitted to the hospital, which might partly account for the increase in fatality, although the hospital throughout most of its history only admitted patients above the age of seven, and most of them appear to have been servants of the subscribers to the hospital.[506] The mean age of smallpox patients during 1836-51 was 17½ years,[507] and this was probably the mean age of patients throughout the eighteenth century, most of whom were probably young servants from the countryside. The case-fatality rate in the hospital would have been higher than outside, as it only admitted the more serious cases, although this would be counter-balanced to some extent by their average age putting them into the minimal risk category.

The increase in the natural virulence of smallpox can be further traced through various local smallpox censuses which were conducted after the 1720s during the rest of the eighteenth and nineteenth centuries.

Case-Fatality Amongst The Unvaccinated In Smallpox Epidemics, 1740-1893

Locality of the Epidemic	Date	Cases	Deaths	Per Cent Fatality
Northampton[508]	1740	899	132	14½
,, [509]	1747	821	126	15½
Salisbury[510]	1753	1244	165	13
Chelmsford[511]	1753	290	95	33
Chester[512]	1774	1385	202	14½
Leeds[513]	1781	462	130	28
Huddersfield and neighbourhood[514]	1783	458	103	22½
Norwich[515]	1819	200	46	23
Sheffield[516]	1887-88	552	274	49½
Dewsbury[517]	1891-92	366	92	25
Warrington[518]	1892-93	68	24	35½
Leicester[519]	1892-93	158	19	12
London[520]	1892-93	409	199	48½
Gloucester[521]	1892-93	768	314	41

As with the smallpox censuses of the 1720s, this Table reveals a considerable amount of variation from place to place in fatality rates at any one point in time; nevertheless, there is an obvious significant long-term trend, with fatality increasing more or less over the whole period. McVail's finding that virulence peaked in the early 1870s is consistent overall with these figures, except that the Sheffield epidemic of 1887-88 seems to have had the highest case-fatality rate recorded for any community survey. The 1892-93 epidemic in the five towns at the end of the Table had an overall fatality rate of 35.4 per cent amongst the unvaccinated (2321 cases, with 822 deaths), which was over twice that found in the censuses of the 1720s, even though fatality had probably begun to decline at the end of the nineteenth century. There is no evidence that this change had anything to do with age incidence, and this can be illustrated by comparing the figures for Aynho earlier quoted with those for the 1887-88 Sheffield epidemic.

Case-Fatality in the Aynho, 1723-24 and Sheffield, 1887-88 Epidemics[22]

Age (Years)	Cases Aynho	Sheffield	Deaths Aynho	Sheffield	Percentage Fatality Aynho	Sheffield
Under 5	28	128	4	66	14.3	51.6
5-10		100		34		34.0
10-15	47	91	4	32	8.5	35.2
15-20		84		53		63.0
20-30	25	98	6	61	24.0	62.2
30+	32	49	11	28	34.4	57.1
Age Unknown		2		—		—
Total	132	552	25	274	18.9	49.6

Overall case-fatality in Sheffield was nearly three times that of that in Aynho, and the Table clearly reveals that this increase was not a function of age; for example, in the 10-20 age group, the case-fatality rate was 8.5 per cent in Aynho and 48.6 per cent in Sheffield. This was an extreme difference, but the smallest difference is still a significant order—in the 30+ age group: 34.4 per cent in Aynho and 57.1 per cent in Sheffield.

Although some of this increase in fatality may have been due to a deterioration in hygiene—particularly when we compare a place like Aynho with somewhere like Sheffield—we saw earlier that the hygiene hypothesis had little to support it. (Also it is likely that overall personal hygiene was better in the last half of the nineteenth century than it was in the eighteenth century.[523]) The most likely explanation of the increase in fatality is that more virulent strains of smallpox were being introduced into the country with the growth of world trade. We have seen that Sarkar and his colleagues found a correlation between the virulence of a virus and its excretion in the throat and urine and this confirmed Dixon's clinical observation about the relationship between severity and infectiousness. With the growth of world trade, virulent viruses would drive out the less virulent ones, although this would not explain the down-turn in fatality at the end of the nineteenth century. This may have been due to more effective inoculation and vaccination programmes in the countries with the higher fatality rates and more virulent viruses. Whatever the explanation for the increase in virulence, the evidence considered on this subject overwhelmingly leads to the conclusion that there was such an increase. The statistical evidence was confirmed by a number of literary accounts, and we may conclude this section of the discussion with a quote from Lettsom, writing in 1805 at the end of the period of greatest interest to this book:

"I think, from my own experience, that the malignity [of smallpox] even in London is augmenting. When I practised here, 35 years ago, one in ten was the calculation; but I think one in six is now a fair proportion."[524]

We must now sum up this discussion of the extent and fatality of smallpox before the introduction of inoculation, which has necessarily involved detailed consideration of a number of complex technical issues. The following conclusion emerges from this discussion: smallpox was a universal disease affecting all members of the population except for a minority of about five per cent who had natural immunity against the disease; fatality varied from place to place, depending in the main on the periodicity of the disease and the resulting age incidence. In the 1720s the case-fatality rate in towns appears to have been of the order of 15½ per cent, and in the countryside where the majority of the population lived, about 24 per cent. These figures cannot be used however as a direct basis for the estimation of smallpox mortality before the introduction of inoculation for two main reasons: (i) evidence that secondary mortality from complications such as broncho-pneumonia and fulminating infantile convulsions would raise the true mortality figure well above this level; (ii) the case-fatality of smallpox was increasing throughout the whole period under consideration. From a demographic point of view, it does not need much imagination to see what would have happened to the population if effective prophylactic measures (inoculation and vaccination) had not been used against smallpox—a disease with a case-fatality rate of about 45 per cent in the 1860-1880 period, which all except five per cent of the population would normally have caught. Merely to contain smallpox mortality to a stable earlier level would have been a considerable achievement in the light of the very significant increase of the virulence of the disease, but smallpox mortality actually declined dramatically during the last third of the eighteenth century. Additionally, the gradual elimination of a disease which appears to have such a significant impact on fertility, is obviously of great demographic importance; this along with the discussion of the decline of smallpox mortality will be dealt with in the next chapter.

In order to complete our discussion of smallpox mortality before the practice of inoculation, it is necessary to analyse the figures of smallpox mortality which emerge from parish registers and the like. Given the difficulties discussed above about reaching a true smallpox mortality figure—in particular the secondary causes of mortality—these figures have to be treated with considerable caution. Also there are two specific problems of using the figures that are available, both hinging on the fact that they are in the main for towns, rather than country areas: (a) the differing age-incidence and probably lower mortality than average resulting; (b) the existence of pest houses and private burials which were not registered in parish registers (this would have been particularly true of market towns). With these major reservations, we can look at all the available figures of registered smallpox mortality in the pre-inoculation period, which in the countryside at large I have taken before the 1760s when the popular Suttonian innovation was introduced, and in some of the larger towns I have assumed extended to the end of the 1770s (it was probably later in the really big towns, but I have attempted to make the more cautious assumption).

The following Table is compiled from statistics which are thought to be reasonably accurate; I have expressed smallpox mortality as a proportion of smallpox deaths per 100 births/deaths, although I have used the ratio per 100 births wherever possible as it more accurately summarizes the proportion of the population (ever born) who were registered as being killed by smallpox. Where population is static, the proportions expressed as a ratio of births or deaths will be the same, but in large towns like London in the eighteenth century the death rate was much higher than the birth rate, and we are more interested in the proportion of young children killed by smallpox, as the disease mainly affected young children in large towns like London and most of the other towns represented in the Table. Where reliable statistics of the number of births are not available, I have expressed smallpox mortality as a proportion of the number of total deaths; for example, according to available statistics about a third of all children born in Dublin between 1715 and 1746 died from smallpox—this is an unusually high proportion, and may be due to the under-registration of births of Roman Catholics who

*Smallpox Mortality Before the Introduction of
Popular Inoculation*

Place and Period	Smallpox Deaths	All Deaths	All Births	Average Annual Smallpox Mortality
Dublin, 1661-90[535]	472 (Annual Average)	2236 (Annual Average)		21 per 100 deaths
Dublin, 1715-46[526]	13,759	74,585		18½ per 100 deaths
Kilmarnock, 1728-62[527]	621		4514	14 per 100 births
London, 1730-39[528]	19,700		170,000	11½ per 100 births
Boston, Lincs., 1749-57[529]	106		691	15½ per 100 births
Maidstone, 1752-61[530]	252		1462	17 per 100 births
Manchester, 1769-74[531]	589	3807		15½ per 100 deaths
Liverpool, 1772-74[532]	662		3559	18½ per 100 births
Chester, 1772-77[533]	369		3970 (1764-73)	15 per 100 births

objected to Anglican rites. The proportion of total deaths due to
smallpox in Dublin (about 20 per cent) is relatively high compared to the statistics of mortality in other places during the
same period—the proportion of total deaths due to smallpox in
London was never much greater than eight per cent during the
same period (1661-1746). This difference could partly be due to
economic and environmental factors, *i.e.* poverty may have raised
smallpox mortality in Dublin, although there is no particular
evidence for this conclusion. An alternative explanation is that
the registration of smallpox deaths was much more accurate in
Dublin than in London, and there is certainly evidence of significant under-registration of smallpox deaths in London. However,
registered smallpox mortality in Dublin was higher than that for
most other places where statistics are available, although there are
examples of apparently higher mortality over a long period of
time; for example, an account was sent to Howlett of smallpox
mortality in Great Chart, Kent, where "its burials in a period of
twenty years immediately subsequent to the revolution [1688-
1707] were 192—but almost 100 of them were occasioned by the
small-pox."[534] There is no mention of deaths from smallpox in
the Great Chart parish register, although the total number of
deaths during the period mentioned according to the register is
192. There is no indication that there was any great epidemic in

the parish during the period, but this does not necessarily mean that the number of smallpox deaths mentioned by Howlett's correspondent did not occur, for there is evidence that smallpox did not always create epidemics but sometimes only produced a few deaths at any one time; for example, Haygarth's statement that "on comparing several neighbouring villages, we observe, some entirely free from the distemper, others have only a few infected, others suffer a general seizure."[535] Nevertheless, the smallpox mortality at Great Chart according to Howlett's account (about 50 per cent of all deaths due to smallpox) was much higher than most known mortality in England during the same period, which leads us to suspect the accuracy of Howlett's correspondent's account. According to the statistics presented, mortality varied between 11½ and 21½ smallpox deaths per 100 births/deaths during the eighteenth century before the introduction of popular inoculation; these statistics also indicate a tendency for smallpox mortality to increase over time and this conforms with the known rise in the case-fatality rate during the same period.

The significance of smallpox mortality before the introduction of popular inoculation is not only depicted by statistical evidence, but is confirmed by literary sources. In the church at Great Barrington, Oxfordshire, there is a monument to the Bray family who were the local gentry:

"Sir Giles Bray married Frances Ashcomb, of Alvescot in Oxfordshire. They had five sons and two daughters, and lost six of them from smallpox. Reginald, the first-born died of smallpox, December 23, 1688; Edmund, died of the same disease when serving as an officer with the Army at the siege of 'Mastrich'. Giles, John, Ashcomb, and Mary, All Dyed also of the same fatal Distemper to this family."[536]

Edmund, who had died at "Mastrich", was the father of two children, Jane and Edward,

"She dyed of the Small Pox at her Aunt Catchmay's in Gloucester, on Monday the One and Twentieth of May 1711 in the Eighth Year of her Age . . . He dyed upon Christmas Day 1720 of the Smallpox at the Royal Academy at Angiers in France, in the Fifteenth year of his age . . ."[537]

This extreme mortality of smallpox was not of course typical at this time, as it was more fatal in some families than others. This is partly reflected in the diary of John Score, a wealthy citizen of Exeter, who recorded the illnesses of his family amongst other things:

"1711—'This summer the Small Pox raged very much in Exeter.' A son had it and recovered (Sept. 15th). 1716, Sept.

7th a daughter had smallpox and recovered—'A great many dyed this season in the Small-Pox.' 1724, Feb. 3. A child had smallpox and recovered. 1724, March 3. A son had smallpox and recovered. 1729, August. A son had smallpox and recovered. 1729, September. Two daughters had smallpox and recovered—'The Small Pox was very fatall to some. Mr Vivian lost all his children, being four sons.' 1731, Feb. A son aged 2 yrs 5 months had 'Small Pox of the confluent kind' and died on the twelfth day."[538]

Of the eight Score children who caught smallpox, only one died—this is to be contrasted to the Vivian family, where all four children caught and died from the disease. It is clear that large numbers of children were dying from smallpox in Exeter, during epidemics which returned every five years or so. There are many examples of a large number of a particular family being wiped out by the disease, and I shall conclude this chapter by quoting one final example reported in Dodsley's Annual Register in 1762:

"The Hon. John Petre, brother to the Lord Petre, who died lately, aged 24, is said to be the eighteenth person of that family that has died of smallpox in 27 years."[539]

CHAPTER 9

The Conquest of Smallpox

It is possible to assess the impact of inoculation on smallpox mortality in particular parishes through the parish register evidence. It is unfortunate that this type of evidence is only rarely available and a disproportionate amount is for large towns which contained only a small minority of the total population during the latter half of the eighteenth century. Because inoculation was practised much more extensively in the countryside than in large towns, the statistics which are most easily available (those for the large towns) give a very misleading picture of the extent of the decline in smallpox mortality. It is partly possible to overcome this problem by: (1) using statistics compiled in connection with general inoculation; and (2) those derived from parish registers when information on smallpox mortality is given. Some of the figures mentioned in the literature in connection with general inoculations do give a number of people dying from smallpox, presumably either those who caught the disease before the general inoculation or exempted themselves from it; for example, in the general inoculation at Northwold, Norfolk in 1788, when 300 people were inoculated, only eleven died from natural smallpox.[540] An even better example, is the general inoculation which took place at Hevingham, Norfolk in 1794:

"In the month of May of this year were inoculated for the Small Pox 3 Adults, 223 under 20 years, and 11 took ye Disease by Natural Infection."[541]

The eleven people catching the natural disease represented only about 4½ per cent of all cases, and assuming a case-fatality rate of about 1 in 5 at this time, over 44 lives were saved by inoculation in this parish. The general inoculation at Hungerford, Berks. in 1794 indicates an even greater saving of life; "about one thousand" were inoculated, "not above two or three of which number died," while "about 20 perished with the natural sort."[542] These figures suggest that about 90 per cent of all cases were inoculated (the 20 dying from smallpox representing 100 cases with a case-fatality rate of 1 in 5) and that about 200 lives were saved. Even when a substantial number of people refused to participate in a general inoculation, the saving of lives through inoculation was very considerable; for example, 59 of 250 unprotected people catching smallpox in Bedford in 1778 died from the disease, so the 1100 people inoculated "within one week" would represent the saving of about 280 lives.[543] Assuming that 339 people would have died (59 + 280) without a majority of the population at risk being protected by inoculation, the actual

number of smallpox deaths (59) represents under fifteen per cent
of the number who would have died without inoculation.

This inoculation at Bedford was considered by Dimsdale
to be unsatisfactory because of the relatively large number of
people not inoculated at the time of the mass inoculation.
Dimsdale was satisfied that "the extensive practice of general
Inoculations in the country, which have prevailed in a remarkable manner . . . has been conducted properly."[544] The result of
inoculating practically all the population at risk was the virtual
extinction of smallpox mortality, as had been achieved in Hertford through Dimsdale's personal efforts. Similarly smallpox was
in effect extinguished from Calne in Wiltshire through the
repetition of general inoculations; 800 people were inoculated in
the year 1793, while there were only six deaths from smallpox
in that year.[545] This elimination of smallpox necessarily followed
from the adoption of Dimsdale's plan, and in a place like Brighton
where all the vulnerable members of the population were inoculated, the only deaths from smallpox were those that preceded
the general inoculation. Most of the examples of general inoculations given in Chapter 5 were probably of this type, and this is
illustrated by the proportion of the total population involved; the
following Table gives the numbers inoculated set alongside the
population size in 1801 (the date of the first National Census),
for those parishes where information on the number of natural
smallpox deaths is not available:

Place	Date of General Inoculation	Numbers Inoculated	Parish Population in 1801 (From Census)
Irthlinborough, Northants.	1778	Above 500	811
Diss, Norfolk	1784	1100	2246
Painswick, Gloucs.	1785	738	3150
		(by G. C. Jenner)	
Brighton, Sussex	1794	2113	5669 (1794 Pop.)
Lewes, Sussex	1794	2890	4909
Dursley, Gloucs.	1797	1475	2379
Tenterden, Kent	1798	1167	2370

Most of these general inoculations involved approximately half
the total population, although in several instances it is even
higher than this. Most of them took place in quite large market
towns, and were probably like Brighton in 1786, having about the
same number of people who had already had smallpox as required
inoculating (in the case of Brighton in 1786, 1733 who had been
through the smallpox, as against 1887 who were inoculated).
Inoculation continued to contribute to the saving of lives during

Smallpox Mortality from Epidemics in Boston, U.S.A. in the Eighteenth Century[516]

	1677-78	1702	1721	1730	1752	1764	1776	1788	1792
Population	4000	6750	10,700	13,500	15,684	15,500			19,300
Natural Smallpox Cases	700		5759	3600	5545	699	304	122	232
Deaths		213	842	500	539	124	29	40	69
Deaths per 1000 cases			146	139	97	177	95	328	298
Inoculated Smallpox Cases			287	400	2124	4977	4988	2121	9152
Deaths			6	12	30	46	28	19	179
Deaths per 1000 cases			21	30	14	9	6	9	20
Total Smallpox Deaths	700	213	848	512	569	170	57	59	284
Deaths per 1000 population	175	32	79	37	36	11	10	6	10
Left the town					1843	1537			262
Escaped disease in town					174	519			221
Had Smallpox before					5998	8200			10,300

the nineteenth century and helped to radically diminish small-pox mortality; for example, during the epidemic in the Chichester region of 1821/22, there were "not more than 130 or 140 cases of natural smallpox" of which number "about twenty proved fatal,"[547] an insignificant number when set against the two to three thousand both inoculated and vaccinated (*i.e.* a total of between four to six thousand).

The second type of statistic referred to earlier—measuring changes in smallpox mortality over time by using parish registers and similar documents—is really the most satisfactory way of assessing the effect of inoculation on smallpox mortality. Ideally, the type of information required to measure the effect of inoculation on mortality is that illustrated in the preceding Table for Boston, U.S.A. during the eighteenth century, such information not being available for anywhere in Britain during the same period.

Three important conclusions may be reached from this Table: (*1*) the overall smallpox death rate was reduced from 175 deaths per 1000 living in 1677-78 to 10 per 1000 by 1792; (*2*) this was achieved in spite of a general increase in the case-fatality rate (about 30 per cent of those catching the natural disease died from it in 1792); (*3*) the reduced mortality may be directly attributed to inoculation, which protected the vast majority of the population at risk from 1764 onwards.

It is unfortunate that similar evidence is not available for Britain during the same period, and it is only possible to quote statistics of smallpox mortality in places where inoculation is known to have been effectively introduced at a certain point of time. The Maidstone parish register contains entries of people dying from smallpox and we know from Howlett's pamphlet on the population and health of the town that popular inoculation was introduced into the town in 1766 when Daniel Sutton conducted a mass inoculation.

Smallpox Mortality at Maidstone, Kent, 1740-1799[548]

Period	Smallpox Deaths	All Deaths	Smallpox Deaths as a Proportion of all Deaths
			%
1740-51	260	1594	16.3
1752-63	202	1616	12.5
1764-75	76	1798	4.2
1776-87	122	1992	6.1
1788-99	31	2308	1.3

These statistics of changing smallpox mortality must not be taken too literally because of the deficiencies and inaccuracies in the registration of death from the disease discussed in an earlier chapter; this point is even more important to keep in mind with statistics derived from parish registers, where the completeness of registration of known deaths from smallpox is uncertain (it is possible that several deaths from smallpox were simply not registered, as registration served no function other than the interest of the incumbent keeping the register). However, these Maidstone statistics do indicate the trend of a marked reduction in smallpox mortality during the latter half of the eighteenth century: that this was due to inoculation is confirmed by Howlett's account of the subject. By the end of the eighteenth century smallpox had disappeared from the register as a cause of death, the last mention of the disease occurring in 1797 when two children were listed as having died from it. Another parish register which lists death from smallpox is that for Calne, Wilts.

Smallpox Deaths in Calne, Wilts., 1703-1802[549]

Period	1703-1722	1723-42	1743-62	1763-82	1783-1802
Number Smallpox Deaths	84	205	122	54	8

This Table suggests that smallpox became more virulent during the period 1723-24 which accords well with the earlier analysis of changes in virulence and case-fatality; however the relatively small number of smallpox deaths during 1703-22 might be due to under-registration. The Table also indicates that smallpox mortality began to decline from the period 1743-62 onwards. The history of inoculation in Calne before 1782 is unknown, but it is known that general inoculations were carried out in the town in 1782 and 1793. The clearest indication of the reduction of smallpox mortality in the town is to compare the epidemic of 1732 when 173 people were registered as dying from smallpox with the numbers dying in the two years of general inoculation (which probably would have become full-blown epidemics without inoculation): ten in 1782 and six in 1793. The scale of the decrease in the number of smallpox deaths between the earlier (1732) and later period (1782-93) is consistent with the known number of inoculations during the latter (over 800 people inoculated during September 1793).

A similar pattern of smallpox mortality to that in Calne is found in Basingstoke, Hants. during the eighteenth century.[550] The first registered epidemic occurred in 1714 when 50 people were listed as dying from smallpox. The next major epidemic occurred in 1741 with 125 registered as dying from the disease; this number is, however, almost certainly an under-statement of the actual number of smallpox deaths as the total number of deaths rose to 220 during that year, whereas the average number of total deaths was 50 for the preceding and following three years—suggesting that there were about 170 smallpox deaths in 1741. No major epidemics of the magnitude of that in 1741 occurred after that date, although 52 people are listed as dying from the disease in 1781. Thirty people are registered as dying from smallpox between 1782 and 1803, the result of one or two people dying every year or so. Nothing is known about the history of inoculation in Basingstoke, but presumably it must have been practised on a fairly extensive scale in order to prevent the recurrence of epidemics of the 1741 type. There is other evidence of the Basingstoke kind, which is suggestive rather than conclusive because of the lack of information about inoculation necessary to interpret the reduction of smallpox mortality.

Smallpox Mortality at Boston, Lincs., 1749-1802[551]

Period	Smallpox Deaths	Baptisms	Smallpox Deaths per 100 Baptisms
			%
1749-75	360	2551	14.1
1776-1802	244	4622	5.25

Smallpox epidemics occurred regularly every seven or eight years in Boston and therefore most deaths would have been of young children. It is therefore appropriate to express smallpox deaths as a proportion of baptisms, and the reduction from about fourteen to five per cent of all children dying of this disease during the latter half of the eighteenth century was a substantial demographic gain. There appears to have been a similar decline in smallpox mortality at Chester. About fifteen per cent of all children born died of smallpox during 1772-77 (369 smallpox deaths 1772-77, 3970 children baptised 1764-73[552]) in the town, and although there is no exactly comparable information for a later date, the parish register of Holy Trinity, Chester, does suggest that there was a marked decline in smallpox mortality after the first period 1772-77. During the period 1787-95 in Holy Trinity, Chester, there were 35 smallpox deaths and 458 baptisms, a ratio of 7.6 smallpox deaths per 100 births, whereas between 1796 and 1802 there were 28 smallpox deaths and 559 baptisms, a ratio of 5 per 100.[553] Holy Trinity was a suburban parish and inhabited by the poorer members of the town, where smallpox mortality would be expected to be greatest because of their slow acceptance of inoculation.[554] Therefore it appears that smallpox mortality fell in the town at least from 15 deaths per 100 children born to 5 per 100.

This decline of smallpox in Chester was associated with the work of Haygarth, who started a society for inoculating the poor in 1780. Haygarth's society also adopted at his instigation a programme of isolating all smallpox cases, so as to stop the spread of the disease, and he later emphasized this aspect of his work because of the difficulty in getting the poor to accept inoculation in Chester. In fact, Haygarth felt there was so much resistance to inoculation that he became rather disillusioned with the proposal for general inoculations in the town, and even went on to argue, like Dimsdale, that partial inoculations could be damaging through spreading the natural form of the disease to unprotected people (this was in spite of his belief that inoculation was only a thirtieth to a fiftieth as infectious as natural smallpox). In 1793, he wrote:

"as far as my circle of observation extends, both in England and Wales, this improved method of communicating the distemper [inoculation] has manifestly appeared to be injurious to the poor, though eminently useful to the rich. It has become prejudicial to the community, though human art never bestowed so valuable a blessing as it confers on the few intelligent individuals who adopt it."[555]

Haygarth made it clear that he mainly had the town areas in mind when he made this statement—we saw earlier how he had stated in 1785 that "whole villages in the neighbourhood (Chester), and many other parts of Britain, have been inoculated with one consent"—but the evidence considered on Chester itself casts considerable doubt on Haygarth's claim. He himself in his book of 1785 gave the following evidence on the recent history of inoculation and smallpox in Chester, quoting from the Report of the Small-Pox Society of Chester, dated Sept. 17, 1782:

"Last spring, 128 poor children were inoculated by the numbers of the Small-pox society; these, added to the 85 inoculated in the spring of 1780, made the whole number 213; during the last four years, 203 private patients have been inoculated: in all four hundred and sixteen . . . Taking the whole period of four years, ending March 30, 1782, the Small-pox has been fatal to 139, or 35 annually . . . whereas the annual average of deaths by the distemper for six years previous to the establishment of the society, was 63."[556]

Given what we know about case-fatality rates at this time, the reduction of smallpox deaths from 63 a year to 35 a year appears to have been entirely due to inoculation, and seems to have been a part of a long-term trend in the reduction of smallpox mortality in Chester. This is not the only evidence to make Haygarth's statement about the damage done by inoculation suspect; smallpox in Chester and other large towns was a young child's disease at this time, which means the disease was endemic. In this situation, it was impossible for inoculation to spread smallpox, as it already universally affected all (young) members of the population (we saw earlier that Dimsdale's argument suffered from the same fallacy in London). The reason for Haygarth's critical attitude towards inoculation appears to have lain in his disappointment at the failure of the policy of general inoculation in Chester and other large towns, along with his passionate belief in the efficacy of isolating smallpox cases so as to contain the disease. This belief seems to have distorted Haygarth's perception and understanding of evidence, which when looked at carefully, goes against the case he was arguing. He gave in his writings examples of places which he considered had been able to avoid smallpox for very long periods by practising a policy of isolation; he quoted a letter from Howlett stating that the three parishes of Boughton, Hunton and Howlett's own native parish in Kent, had only had 10 smallpox deaths in the twenty-year period 1762-82,[557] but failed to mention Howlett's descriptions of general inoculations in the area. Similarly, he quoted in 1793 the secretary of the local Chester infirmary on the absence of smallpox in Sussex as follows:

> "Mr Connah, secretary of the infirmary, and formerly inspector of the small-pox society at Chester, informs me that both the casual and inoculated distemper are carefully avoided in Sussex. He was a practical surgeon at Seaford in that county . . . The town contains about seven hundred people. He was informed, that, about eleven years ago, one person had died of the small-pox, but could not learn when a like misfortune had happened in the place, antecendent to that period."[558]

We are in a fortunate position with which to evaluate this statement of Haygarth's, as East Sussex was one of the areas which was covered fairly intensively for the present book. We have seen earlier from the letters of Thomas Davies, bailiff to the Glynde estate, and from evidence coming out of general inoculation in places like Lewes and Brighton, that people in Sussex did indeed fear and avoid smallpox as much as possible—but once an epidemic had begun to establish itself, inoculation was rapidly resorted to. Haygarth singled out Seaford as a particular example of a town that had managed to avoid smallpox, yet Davies tells us in one of his letters, that Seaford "are inclined to our scheme" of general inoculation.[559] We do not know whether Seaford did actually carry out such a general inoculation (the relevant local historical records have disappeared), but given that everywhere else in East Sussex was doing so, it is likely that they did as well; whatever happened at Seaford, it is clear that Haygarth gave his readers a very misleading impression when he wrote that "the casual and inoculated distemper are carefully avoided in Sussex."

It is not only statements of the kind made by Haygarth which have misled historians about the role of inoculation, but also the reliance of certain key statistics—those based on the London Bills of Mortality—which have been quoted, repeatedly, in various writings on the subject. At the outset it must be said that the reliability of these statistics is likely to be very low indeed, as recent research has indicated that often a majority of vital events could escape registration.[560] Additionally, as with all statistics, the way they are arranged and interpreted can completely alter the conclusions reached from them; most nineteenth century writers on this subject were supporters of vaccination and opponents of the old inoculation, and used the London statistics to show that smallpox mortality had not declined through the use of inoculation, but on the contrary, they argued, the disease had been maintained through secondary contagion. The basic fallacy of this argument—that a disease cannot be spread (from the point of view of overall mortality) in a place like London, where smallpox was endemic and more-or-less confined to children "under the age of seven"—seems to have escaped all nineteenth century writers, both those for and against inoculation. One later writer less hostile to inoculation that most—Dr George Gregory—argued that inoculation did reduce smallpox mortality in London, from 65,383 deaths in 1711-40 to 63,308 in 1741-70 and 57,268 in 1771-1800[561] Gregory seems to have been unaware that the fairly rapid increase in London's population during this period would have increased the number of susceptibles (i.e. young children vulnerable to smallpox), and that to get a true measure of changing mortality it would be necessary to express the number of deaths as a proportion of the number of children. In the following Table, I give the numbers of smallpox burials, baptisms and the percentage of burials per 100 baptisms, the latter being an attempt to allow for a change in the number at risk.

Smallpox Mortality in London, 1740-1829[562]

Period	Smallpox Burials	Baptisms	Smallpox burials per 100 baptisms
	(nearest 100)	(nearest 1000)	%
1740-49	20,000	146,000	13.7
1750-59	19,600	147,000	13.3
1760-69	22,000	159,000	13.8
1770-79	22,100	173,000	12.1
1780-89	17,100	177,000	9.6
1790-99	16,600	187,000	8.9
1800-09	13,700	199,000	6.9
1810-19	8,500	221,000	3.8
1820-29	7,000	257,000	2.7

This Table indicates that smallpox mortality fell in London after 1769 until the 1820s when it was a fifth of what it had been during the 1760s and before. The fall was relatively gradual, spread over a long period of time, which fits with the chronology of the spread of inoculation (and vaccination after 1800). These London statistics are only suggestive of the trend of mortality over time, and obviously not too much reliance can be placed on the magnitude of changes because of the unreliability of the raw data, as well as the various sources of under-registration of the true mortality from smallpox discussed earlier. Inoculation cannot be said to have nearly eliminated smallpox in London as it did in a place like Maidstone and other provincial towns and villages, although inoculation was practised very extensively in London up until at least 1840, by which time the disease was well under control. Therefore it would appear that inoculation significantly contributed to the reduction of smallpox mortality during the period 1770-1840, no mean feat at a time when the disease was greatly increasing in virulence.

In addition to this more systematic statistical evidence, there is other somewhat piecemeal information to suggest that the disease had all but disappeared in the country at large by the end of the eighteenth and beginning of the nineteenth centuries. In 1776 Dimsdale summarized the effect of inoculation in the town of Hertford as follows:

". . . within these [last] ten years not six persons have died in Hertford of this disease [smallpox]; whereas before the practice [of inoculation] was so generally adopted, the Small Pox has frequently been epidemic and destroyed a great number of inhabitants . . ."[563]

The historian of Tamworth, Staffs., also noted the effect of inoculation on mortality and population in the town:

"Hence, it is evident that a very considerable increase took place in the population of the parish, particularly during the last ten years [of the eighteenth century] . . . The number of baptisms also became more disproportionate to the burials. This was attributed [by the Rev. F. Blick] to the better mode adopted for preserving the lives of infants, when inoculation began generally to prevail."[564]

In the Milton Ernest, Beds. parish register the cause of death is given for the years 1783-99, during which period smallpox accounted for only one of the 150 deaths,[565] an insignificant proportion at a time when the average case-fatality rate of the disease was probably twenty per cent and above. Similarly at Horton Kirbie, Kent, a village with a population of about 400 people, there were only six smallpox deaths between 1772 and 1810[566] and at Whittington, Salop., with a population of about 1300, nineteen children died from smallpox in 1775-76, two in 1785, after which there were no more mentions of smallpox deaths.[567] At Selattyn, Salop., the number of smallpox burials between 1784-1812 (when the cause of all deaths was recorded) was nineteen and the number of baptisms 778, yielding a smallpox mortality rate of about 2.5 smallpox deaths per hundred births. This very low mortality was not due to the infrequency or absence of smallpox as sixteen of the nineteen deaths took place amongst children under the age of ten years and only one of them was that of an adult.[568] Inoculation was almost certainly responsible for the very low smallpox mortality in this village after 1784. At Luton, Beds., there were only 11 smallpox deaths out of a total of 1694 during 1800-12—this low mortality could have been due to the introduction of vaccination but we have seen that there was a very successful general inoculation in the town in 1788 which it was intended to repeat annually.

The literary evidence provides abundant confirmation of the impact of inoculation on smallpox mortality. The decline of smallpox and the resulting increase in population was first commented upon by a contributor to the satirical periodical *The World* in 1755:

"The world, in general . . . is certainly much over-peopled . . . This inconvenience had in great measure been hitherto prevented, by the proper number of people who were daily removed by the smallpox in the natural way; **one**, at least, in **seven** dying, to the great ease and convenience of the survivors; whereas since inoculation has prevailed, all hopes of thinning out people that way are entirely at an end; not above **one** in **three hundred** being taken off, to the great encumbrance of society."[569]

The writer of this satirical piece appears to have mainly had "worthy country gentlemen" and their families in mind, for he goes on to describe how they were deserting the countryside for the metropolis where they no longer had anything to fear from smallpox because of inoculation. Nearly twenty years later, Goldsmith included another humorous reference to inoculation in his play *She Stoops to Conquer*, written in 1773, Mrs Hardcastle saying to Hastings:

"I vow, since Inoculation began, there is no such thing to be seen as a plain woman. So one must dress a little particular, or one may escape in the crowd."[570]

Obviously this is not the most reliable form of evidence, but it does suggest that smallpox was beginning to disappear amongst the wealthy and fashionable classes. More reliable evidence of this change is to be found in reports sent to Haygarth which he discussed in his book published in 1793:

"Several respectable Correspondents have declined to give a decided opinion on this subject [of smallpox], from want of opportunity to make observations in their own practice. A physician of the greatest eminence both in rank and erudition gives the following very sufficient reason for his silence on this point. 'In London we have very few opportunities of seeing the smallpox. For the last five and twenty years, the number of variolous patients, who have fallen under my care, is very inconsiderable.' Another distinguished physician and author in a large city says, 'I have not seen six private patients in the smallpox in eighteen years . . .'."[571]

Clearly, this would only apply to the wealthy who were the employers of the "private" and "distinguished" physicians. Nevertheless it does suggest that smallpox had virtually disappeared as a disease amongst the wealthy classes by about 1770, which according to other evidence already discussed can only have been due to the practice of inoculation.

The first person to discuss at any length in print the effect of inoculation on smallpox mortality and general population was the Rev. John Howlett, who wrote on many economic and demographic subjects. Howlett was Vicar of Great Dunmow, Essex, for many years and was resident in Maidstone, Kent at different times. He was in a particularly good position to know about the effects of inoculation in the country as a whole as a result of his demographic studies. In September 1782 he described in the *Gentleman's Magazine* the nature of an enquiry he was engaged in:

". . . during the last twelve months I have sent out between 3 and 4000 written letters and printed papers to the clergy in different parts of the kingdom, in which I have ventured to solicit not only register extracts for different periods in their respective parishes, but likewise, wherever conveniently attainable, actual surveys of the people, together with many curious, perhaps important information."[572]

Included in this "important information" were references to inoculation, an example of which Howlett quoted in a book by him published in 1781:

"A striking instance to the same purpose in the parish of Great Chart, near Ashford in the county of Kent, has been sent me. Its burials in a period of twenty years immediately subsequent to the revolution [1688-1708] were 192—but almost 100 of them were occasioned by the small-pox; whereas in 20 years beginning with 1760, there appears to have been only 4 or 5 who died of that disorder. This diminution my ingenious correspondent imputes to inoculation, and adds 'that no register can, as yet, properly inform us of the thousands that have been preserved by this salutary practice for these 20 years past all over the kingdom . . .'."[573]

In the same publication, Howlett summarized the position on the effects of inoculation as he understood it:

". . . the diminished mortality of . . . provincial towns and villages . . . appears to be chiefly owing to the salutary practice of inoculation . . . where two or three hundred used to be carried [off by smallpox] to their graves in the course of a few months, there are now perhaps not above 20 or 30."[574]

Howlett reached this conclusion before making his more extensive enquiry into population during 1781-82, some of the results of which were published anonymously in a pamphlet by him on changes in the population and health of the town of Maidstone, Kent. This was published in 1782 and Howlett summarized his conclusions *vis-à-vis* smallpox, inoculation and population in Maidstone as follows:

"Upon casting an eye over the annual lists of burials we see, that, before the modern improved practice of inoculation [the Suttonian method] was introduced, every five or six years the average number was almost doubled; and it was found upon enquiry, that at such intervals nearly the smallpox used to repeat its dreadful periodical visits . . . in the short space of 30 years it deprived the town of between five and six hundred of its inhabitants; whereas in the 15 or 16 years that have elapsed since that general inoculation [in 1766] it has occasioned the deaths of only about 60. Ample and satisfactory evidence of the vast benefit the town has received from the salutary invention! And it appears, with a high degree of probability upon proofs similar to the above, that, from the same causes, in the kingdom at large not less than 4 or 500,000 lives were lost in the former of the periods now stated, and that nearly half that number had been saved in the latter . . . This [diminution of the death rate in Maidstone] may . . . be ascribed . . . principally and chiefly to that distinguished blessing of providence, inoculation."[575]

According to Howlett, the radical decline in smallpox mortality in Maidstone after 1766 due to the use of inoculation, was characteristic of many other parts of the country, in most "provincial towns and villages."[576]

During the last twenty years of the eighteenth century it was very common for non-medical writers to note the role of inoculation in radically reducing smallpox mortality and therefore leading to population expansion; for example, Arthur Young the agriculturalist wrote in 1781:

"In several of these parishes where population had for some
periods been rather on the decrease, a great change has
taken place lately, and the last ten years are found to be in a
rapid state of progression; as considerable drains of men
have been made from almost every parish in the kingdom for
the public service in that period, I should not have expected
this result, and know nothing to which it can be owing,
unless the general prevalence of inoculation, which certainly
has been attended with a very great effect."[577]

There are also references to the effects of inoculation on mortality
in the reports on agriculture to the Board of Agriculture at the
end of the eighteenth century. Plymley of Shropshire wrote
before the end of the century:

"I may further add, that since the year 1782, when these
observations were made, the population of this parish has
been increasing: most certainly the inoculation for the
smallpox . . . has been most essential to population throughout this kingdom."[578]

Similarly John Holt of Lancashire wrote in 1795:

"One reason why persons in large manufacturies in Lancashire do not frequently die in great numbers . . . is that they
have (in general) been inoculated in their infancy. Inoculation is the most effectual of all expedients for preserving the
short-lived race of men—many gentlemen pay for the inoculation of the children of the poor in their own neighbourhood."[579]

These observations on the effect of inoculation were made in
passing, as most writers on agriculture did not consider the
causes of population increase as relevant to their subject. This
makes the evidence of Plymley and Holt all the more impressive,
as it was unsolicited and cannot be explained as a function of
partisan interest; both writers agreed that inoculation was very
important in their counties in diminishing smallpox mortality
and increasing population.

I have previously discussed and quoted at length from
Heysham's account of inoculation in the Carlisle Bills of Mortality. He summarized the effect of inoculation on mortality and
population as follows:

"Inoculation, I am persuaded, has also greatly contributed
to the increase of population, not only in Carlisle, but likewise in the whole county of Cumberland. In the year 1779,
when the lower class of inhabitants [of Carlisle] were extremely averse to this salutary discovery, no fewer than
ninety persons died of the natural smallpox; whereas only
151 have died during the eight succeeding years; which is,

upon average, not quite nineteen in each year; and yet the disorder prevailed in every one of these years . . ."[580]

This summary is a useful overall picture of the scale of the effect of inoculation on smallpox mortality in Cumberland; the figures of smallpox cannot be taken too literally as evidence for the decline of mortality, as the particular years discussed may have been untypical, and 1779 may have been a particularly fatal year. The statistics quoted are valuable however for illustrating Heysham's belief about the impact of inoculation on smallpox mortality in the Carlisle area, an effect which was general to the whole of Cumberland.

The impact of inoculation on smallpox mortality and population was noted not only at the local and county level, but also for the country as a whole. A contributor to the *Gentleman's Magazine* argued in the February 1796 edition:

"The increase of people within the last 25 years is visible to every observer . . . Inoculation is the mystic spell that has produced this wonder. Some time between 1738 and 1743 (I speak from memory), the small-pox was so severe at St Edmundsbury, that the assizes were twice, if not three times, held at Ipswich; which supposes a continuation of 18 months. During that term, it was said, that the town had been deprived of a sixth part of its inhabitants: there were no markets, and the town was avoided as the seat of death and terror. This was no more than a common calamity at that time . . . so that it may be safely asserted, that this malady [smallpox], added to the general laws of nature, did at the least equipoize population . . . It is now 30 years since the Suttons, and others under their instructions, had practised their skill in inoculation upon half the kingdom, and had reduced the risk of death to the chance of one in 2000. Hence the great increase of people . . ."[581]

This general statement is all the more convincing for being based on personal experience and observation, although it suffers from being too impressionistic, particularly with reference to the effects of inoculation on population growth. A similar type of statement was made by a contributor to the *Gentleman's Magazine* in 1803, which I have quoted at the very beginning of this book. A part of this statement—concerning the "saving of lives" through inoculation—was questioned by the Editor of the Magazine in a footnote: "On this head Doctors materially differ."[582] The Editor was referring to the criticisms levelled against inoculation by the medical supporters of vaccination, based on abstract a priori medical arguments—that it gave rise to secondary contagion—and it is these criticisms which have led medical historians subsequently to neglect the empirical study of the role of inoculation in the diminution of smallpox mortality. The contributor to the *Gentleman's Magazine* in 1803 was not to be misled by theoretical objections and replied to the Editor's footnote at length in the next edition:

"Of the proportion of deaths in the Natural Small Pox, I have had ocular demonstration, both in the North and West of England, more especially in country villages, the miseries of our large cities and towns . . . Of the great success of Inoculation with the matter of the Small-Pox, I have read some accounts; but have had many more from various medical gentlemen; of whom, some have visited Ireland professedly for that purpose, and others have formed establishments in various parts of the kingdom. A gentleman, of but little medical knowledge, was, some years since, established in this peculiar branch of the profession, who was in the habit of inoculating whole parishes, at a very moderate stated price. It is scarce 20 years since I first became acquainted with some of the family; at which time, they had inoculated near 15,000 persons, mostly in villages and small towns, and in a few years afterwards the number was considerably more than 20,000. From persons well acquainted with the practice, it was agreed, that not one in a thousand of their patients miscarried. This was on the very boundry of Wilts. and Hants., and is well known to every person then resident in its vicinity . . ."[583]

The substance of this correspondent's argument was that nearly everyone caught smallpox before the introduction of inoculation and of these between a fifth and a quarter died; due to inoculation, which became very widespread, only one of every 1000 persons died (after inoculation), leading to an enormous saving of lives, sufficiently great to explain the increase in population during the latter half of the eighteenth century. Again this argument has the advantage of being based on personal experience and observation, but also lacks any detailed statistical estimate of the significance of reduced smallpox mortality on population growth.

These contemporary writers were unaware of course that disease could indirectly effect fertility as well as mortality; I have already discussed the work of Phadke and his colleagues which would lead us to expect smallpox to have had a significant impact on the history of fertility. Reliable figures on changes in fertility among the general population are not available for the relevant period, but T. H. Hollingsworth in his monograph on the demography of the British Peerage has calculated figures for fertility from the sixteenth century onwards. He has summarized the conclusions relevant to the present argument as follows:

"... fertility of the cohorts born between 1550 and 1724 apparently fell from nearly 5 children per married adult to only $3\frac{1}{2}$ ... Hence it would appear that from about 1590 to about 1740 there was a fairly steady decline in fertility ... the trend was arrested (say 1740) ... [and] mean family size rose from $3\frac{1}{2}$ to almost 5 again between ... 1740 and 1815."[584]

This historical pattern of fertility seems to coincide almost exactly with that of smallpox mortality; up until 1740 or thereabouts, smallpox mortality was increasing as a result of the growth in the virulence of the disease, and for the aristocracy who adopted inoculation earlier than the general population, smallpox mortality probably fell from the 1740s onwards. The increasing mortality of the disease up to 1740 would influence fertility as the more severe forms of smallpox would probably have created a greater number of focal lesions in the epidydimis; this would be analogous to severer types of smallpox producing larger crops of skin lesions. After 1740, with the practice of inoculation, the frequency of the focal lesions in the epididymis would decline, and fertility would gradually increase. We would expect to find from Phadke's findings that childlessness grew during the period of increasing smallpox mortality, and Hollingsworth's figures do show an increase for both men and women from about fourteen per cent in the middle of the seventeenth century to about twenty-three per cent by 1740, after which it declines to eighteen or nineteen per cent at the end of the century.[585] There is a certain degree of uncertainty about the reliability of these figures on childlessness, and it appears from Phadke's work that the focal lesions produced by smallpox both reduce the degree of fertility through bringing about oligospermia (both severe and moderate), as well as creating infertility through azoospermia.[586] The extent to which this analysis of smallpox and fertility is applicable to the general population is unknown; at the present we lack sufficiently reliable figures to come to any firm conclusions.

Returning to the problem of the reduction of smallpox mortality, the first national figures for England and Wales only become available after 1837 with the introduction of civil registration. Given what we know about the case-fatality rate of smallpox at this time, it is possible to use the civil registration figures to reach firm conclusions about the effectiveness of prophylactic measures at this time. Both inoculation and vaccination were still being practised, and as they were both variants of the same operation—the inoculation of smallpox virus (with vaccination being the more attenuated form)—it is appropriate to evaluate their joint effectiveness. As about 75 per cent of all smallpox deaths in England and Wales in 1839 occurred in children under five (about 87 per cent under ten),[587] it is again most appropriate to express smallpox mortality as a proportion of births. Smallpox deaths accounted for approximately 1½ per cent of all children born in England and Wales during 1838-44,[588] and this was the highest smallpox mortality ratio recorded under civil registration (*i.e.* mortality ratios were even lower in subsequent periods).[589] This level of mortality was of course insignificant compared to some of the ratios for the pre-inoculation period. In Ireland during the 1830s, smallpox mortality was as low as 2.2 smallpox deaths per 100 births,[590] and this was almost certainly achieved primarily through inoculation rather than vaccination, because at this time "a large proportion of the peasantry in the country parts" were "in favour of inoculation,"[591] and it was in the large majority living in the countryside that smallpox was at its lowest, as can be seen in the following Table.

Smallpox Mortality in Ireland, 1831-40[592]

	Smallpox Deaths (1831-40)	Population (1841)	Annual Average Smallpox Deaths per Million Living
Civic Districts	12,418	1,135,465	1093
Rural Districts	45,459	7,039,659	647

The lower mortality in the rural districts was not a function of the proportion of the population catching the disease, as smallpox was a young child's disease in Ireland at this time—about 49,000 of the total 58,000 smallpox deaths occurred under the age of five[593]—and in both types of area most children had either been inoculated or vaccinated, or caught the disease by the age of five. The total smallpox mortality rate for Ireland during 1831-40 was 710 annual deaths per million living (1841), a very low mortality compared with that for the pre-inoculation period; for example, in Dublin during 1661-90 there were about 8600 smallpox deaths per million living.[594]

Smallpox mortality for both Ireland and England and Wales was insignificant when set alongside the case-fatality rate of the disease. We have already seen that this lay somewhere between the 23 per cent in the Norwich 1819 epidemic and the 49½ per cent for the 1887-88 Sheffield one; smallpox epidemics on the Continent during this period yielded similar levels: 57½ per cent of all unvaccinated cases in the 1828 Digne (France) epidemic were fatal, and of the 10,246 unprotected people who caught smallpox in Milan during 1830-51, 38.3 per cent died.[595] This latter figure refers to the two decades for which the civil registration figure of smallpox mortality in England and Wales was calculated, and given the large numbers on which it is based, it is an appropriate statistic with which to evaluate that mortality (it is also what would be expected from the trend of British case-fatality figures). Thus only 1½ per cent of all children born in England and Wales died of smallpox in 1838-44, when the case-fatality rate was 38.3 per cent. Given that smallpox was a universal disease which had affected everyone even before the advent of inoculation, except for a five per cent minority with natural immunity, the saving of life revealed by these figures is obvious. Without prophylactic measures against smallpox, something like between a quarter and a third of the population would have died directly from smallpox in the post-civil registration period. In addition to this, many more people would have died from secondary broncho-pneumonia and other complicating diseases, and fertility would have been depressed to a significantly reduced level. It is no exaggeration to say that inoculation and vaccination prevented the decimation of the population of the kind that Europe suffered in the fourteenth century onwards, and instead of the rapidly expanding economy of the nineteenth century which we label the Industrial Revolution, there would have been a very prolonged period of decline and stagnation. Inoculation and vaccination were developed through folk medicine and accidental discovery, but they were medical measures completely unrivalled in their impact on health and mortality in the whole history of medicine.

APPENDIX

In an earlier book [*Edward Jenner's Cowpox Vaccine: The History of a Medical Myth* (Caliban Books, 1977)], I have argued that the main stock of Jenner's vaccine was derived not from cowpox, but from smallpox. I attempt to demonstrate that this vaccine originated from virus sent by Woodville to Jenner, and that the contamination with smallpox took place at the end of January 1799 when it was first used in the London Smallpox Hospital. Since writing the book, I have come across further evidence that Jenner relied almost exclusively on Woodville's supply of vaccine, in spite of occasionally having access to other sources. On the 24th February, 1801, Jenner wrote the following letter to Benjamin Waterhouse:

". . . I have sent you also some virus from a new stock, the history of which you shall hear. The old stock, now in use, nearly three years, has not lost any of its original properties, nor do I suppose it ever will. A medical gentleman at Milan, Dr Sacco, who informed me he has inoculated 8000 persons in that city, has lately sent me vaccine virus, taken from a dairy on the plains of Lombardy. It had produced again and again the perfect pustule here. I always ventured to predict, that the cow-pox was not confined to this island only . . . "
[Benjamin Waterhouse, *Information Respecting the Origin, Progress and Efficacy of the Kine Pock Inoculation* (Cambridge, Mass., U.S.A., 1810).]

The old stock of vaccine that Jenner referred to had been sent to Waterhouse in the summer of 1800, and was almost certainly responsible for an outbreak of smallpox in Marblehead, near Boston. Jenner stated that it had been in use nearly three years, and as he wrote this on the 24th February 1801, this meant the vaccine must have been in use before the 24th February 1799. The only successful vaccine used by Jenner or anyone else in this period was that supplied by Woodville. His vaccine was only just over two years old, but Jenner is known to have exaggerated evidence where it suited his purposes, and the above letter is therefore further confirmation of Jenner's reliance on Woodville's vaccine. Although Jenner does refer in the letter to use of Sacco's vaccine, he made it clear to the Royal College of Physicians committee on vaccination in 1807, that he continued to use "Matter that was taken from the cow in 1799", *i.e.* Woodville's contaminated vaccine.

BIBLIOGRAPHY

This bibliography includes only the important sources repeatedly used in this study, which the reader might fruitfully read for further study of the subject treated by the book. Other sources may be found in the footnotes

[P=Pamphlet]

Manuscript Sources
1. *Report and Evidence of the Royal College of Physicians of London on Vaccination* (1807) in the Library of the Royal College of Physicians in London.
2. *Inoculation Letters* in the Royal Society Library.

Printed Sources
PRIMARY:
1. W. Buchan, *Domestic Medicine* (Edinburgh 1769).
2. T. Dimsdale, *Thoughts on General and Partial Inoculation* (1776). [P]
3. T. Dimsdale, *Observations on the Introduction to the Plan of the Dispensary for General Inoculation* (1778). [P]
4. T. Dimsdale, *Tracts on Inoculation* (1781). [P]
5. J. Forbes, "Some Account of the Small-Pox Lately Prevalent in Chichester and its Vicinity", *London Medical Repository*, XIIX (1822).
6. *The Gentleman's Magazine*, 1733-1806.
7. J. Haygarth, *An Inquiry How to Prevent the Small Pox* (Chester 1785).
8. J. Haygarth, *A Sketch of a Plan to Exterminate the Casual Small-Pox* (1793).
9. J. Heysham, "An Abridgement of the Observations on the Bills of Mortality in Carlisle, from the year 1779 to 1787, inclusive", in W. Hutchinson, *The History of Cumberland* (1794).
10. R. Houlton, *Indisputable Facts Relative to the Suttonian Art of Inoculation* (Dublin 1768). [P]
11. J. Howlett, *An Examination of Dr Price's Essay on the Population of England and Wales* (Maidstone 1781). [P]
12. J. Howlett, *Observations on the Increased Population . . . of Maidstone* (Maidstone 1782). [P]
    This pamphlet was published anonymously and an original copy is to be found in Maidstone Museum Library.
13. E. Jenner, *An Inquiry into the Causes and Effects of . . . the Cow Pox* (1798). [P]
14. J. Jurin, *An Account of the Success of Inoculating the Small Pox in Great Britain* (4 Editions, 1724-27). [P]

161

15. J. C. Lettsom, *A Letter to Sir R. Barker . . . and G. Stacpole . . . Upon General Inoculation* (1778). [P]
16. J. C. Lettsom, *An Answer to Baron Dimsdale's Review of Dr Lettsom's Observation on the Baron's Remarks respecting a Letter upon General Inoculation* (1779). [P]
17. Alexander Monro, "Account of the Inoculation of Small Pox in Scotland (1765)", in A. Monro (ed.), *The Works of Alexander Monro M.D.* (Edinburgh 1781).
18. J. Moore, *History of Small-Pox and Vaccination* (1815).
19. T. J. Pettigrew, *Memoirs of the Life and Writings of the late John Coakley Lettsom*, 2 (1817).
20. J. G. Scheuchzer, *An Account of the Success of Inoculating the Small Pox in Great Britain* (1729). [P]
21. Sir J. Sinclair (ed.), *The Statistical Account of Scotland*, 21 Vols. (Edinburgh 1791-99).
22. T. Short, *A History of the Air, Weather, Seasons, etc.* (1749).
23. T. Short, *New Observations on Bills of Mortality* (1751).
24. J. Watkinson, *An Examination of a Charge brought against Inoculation* (1777). [P]
25. W. Woodville, *The History of the Inoculation of the Small-Pox in Great Britain* (1796).

SECONDARY:
1. C. Creighton, *The History of Epidemics* (Cambridge 1897), 2.
2. C. W. Dixon, *Smallpox* (1962).
3. W. R. Clayton Heslop, "Notes on the History, Incidence and Treatment of Smallpox in Norfolk", *Norfolk Archaeology*, XXX (1952).
4. D. V. Glass and D. E. C. Eversley (Eds), *Population in History* (1965).
5. T. H. Hollingsworth, "The Demography of the British Peerage", *Population Studies*, Supplement (November 1964).
6. G. Miller, *The Adoption of Inoculation for Smallpox in England and France* (1957).
7. *Royal Commission On Vaccination*, 6 Reports—Final Report (1889-1896).

REFERENCES

1. See *The Lancet*, January 1st, 1977, p. 26; *The Lancet*, February 12th, 1977, pp. 352, 354.
2. *Gentleman's Magazine*, LXXIII, i (1803), p. 213.
3. T. H. Hollingsworth, "The Demography of the British Peerage", Supplement to *Population Studies*, *18*, 2, p. 57.
4. P. E. Razzell, "Population Change in Eighteenth Century England: a Re-Appraisal" in Michael Drake (Ed), *Population in Industrialization* (1969), p. 134.
5. "Reports of John Finlainson on the Evidence and Elementary Facts on which the Tables of Life Annuities are Founded", *Parliamentary Papers*, 1829 (3).
6. Peter Razzell, *Edward Jenner's Cowpox Vaccine: The History of a Medical Myth* (1977).
7. J. Z. Holwell, *An Account of the Manner of Inoculation for the Smallpox on the East Indies* (1767), p. 16.
8. *Ibid*, p. 20.
9. Perrot Williams, "Part of two Letters concerning a Method of procuring the Small Pox, used in South Wales", *Philosophical Transactions*, 31-32 (1720-23), p. 262.
10. Richard Wright, "A Letter on the same Subject, from Mr Richard Wright, Surgeon of Haverford West, to Mr Sylvanus Bevan, Apothecary in London", *Philosophical Transactions*, 31-32 (1720-23), p. 267.
11. *Ibid*, pp. 268, 269.
12. Emanuel Timoni, "An Account, or History, of the Procuring the Small Pox by Incision; or Inoculation. As it has for Some Time Been Practised at Constantinople", *Philosophical Transactions*, XXIX (April-June 1714), pp. 72-82.
13. *Ibid*.
14. *Ibid*.
15. *Ibid*.
16. *Ibid*.
17. Peter Kennedy, *An Essay on External Remedies* (1715), p. 155.
18. Dr Jacob Pylarinus, "Nova et tuta excitandi per transplatationem methodus; nuper inventa et in usum tracta", *Philosophical Transactions*, XXIX (Jan.-Mar. 1716), pp. 393-99.
19. Quoted in C. W. Dixon, *Smallpox* (1962), pp. 219, 220.
20. Charles Maitland, *An Account of Inoculating the Smallpox* (1723), p. 7.
21. "Letter From P. Russel", *Philosophical Transactions*, Vol. 58 (1768), p. 142.
22. W. Wagstaffe, M.D., *A Letter to Dr Friend Shewing the Danger and Uncertainty of Inoculating the Smallpox* (1722).
23. James Jurin, M.D., "A Letter to the Learned Dr Caleb Cotesworth, F.R.S.", *Philosophical Transactions*, 31-32 (1720-23), p. 224.

24. James Porter, "Queries sent to a Friend in Constantinople, by Dr Maty, F.R.S., and answered by His Excellency James Porter", *Philosophical Transactions*, 49 (1755-56), p. 104.

25. Emanuel Timoni, "Extract of a Letter Communicated to the Royal Society by Samuel Horseman, M.D.", *Philosophical Transactions*, Vol. 38 (1734), pp. 646, 647.

26. Maitland, *op. cit.*, pp. 8-10.

27. *Ibid*, p. 24.

28. Wagstaffe, *op. cit.*, p. 25.

29. *Ibid*, pp. 30, 31.

30. See for example Maitland, *op. cit.* pp. 14, 18; Wagstaffe, *op. cit.*

31. Thomas Nettleton, M.D., "A Letter to Dr Jurin", *Philosophical Transactions*, 31-32 (1720-23), p. 38.

32. Joseph Rogers, *An Essay on Epidemic Diseases* (1734), p. 180.

33. J. G. Scheuchzer, *An Account of the Success of Inoculating the Small-Pox* (1729), p. 24.

34. Henry Newman, "The way of proceeding in the small pox inoculated in New England", *Philosophical Transactions*, 31-32 (1720-23), p. 31.

35. Zabdiel Boylston, *An Historical Account of the Small-Pox Inoculated in New England* (London, 1726), p. 50.

36. "Letter from Claudius Amyand, Esqr., Segt. Surgeon, dated Janr. 16th, 1724", *Inoculation Letters*, MSS 245 (In), in the Royal Society Library. Hereafter referred to as *Inoculation Letters*.

37. Lady Mary Wortley Montagu, "A Plain Account of the Inoculating of the Small Pox by a Turkey Merchant", *Journal of the History of Medicine*, Vol. 8 (1953), p. 402.

38. Sir Hans Sloane, "An Account of Inoculation by Sir Hans Sloane, Bart., given to Mr Ranby, to be published, Anno 1736. Communicated by Thomas Birch, D.D., Secret. Royal Society", *Philosophical Transactions*, 49 (1755-56), pp. 519, 520.

39. James Burges, *An Account of the Preparation and Management Necessary to Inoculation* (1764), pp. 35, 36.

40. Henry Barnes, M.D., "Note on an Autograph Letter describing Inoculation of Small-Pox in Carlisle in 1755", *Proceedings of the Royal Society of Medicine*, 9, No. 2 (1916), p. 21.

41. Barnes, *op. cit.*, p. 22.

42. "Robert Sutton's Advertisement", *Ipswich Journal*, 1st May, 1762.

43. "Robert Sutton's Advertisement", *Ipswich Journal'* 25th September, 1762.

44. Robert Houlton, *The Tryal of Mr Daniel Sutton for the High Crime of Preserving the Lives of His Majesty's Liege Subjects by Means of Inoculation* (1767), p. 7.

45. Robert Houlton, *A Sermon . . . in Defence of Inoculation* (1767), pp. 39, 40.
46. Daniel Sutton, *The Inoculator, or Suttonian System of Inoculation* (1796), p. 77.
47. Thomas Dimsdale, *The Present Method of Inoculating for the Small-Pox* (1767), pp. 24, 25.
48. William Bromfield, *Thoughts Arising from Experience Concerning the Present Peculiar Method of Treating Persons Inoculated for the Small-Pox* (1767), p. 14.
49. W. R. Clayton Heslop, "Notes on the History, Incidence and Treatment of Smallpox in Norfolk", *Norfolk Archaeology*, XXX (1952), p. 6.
50. *Ibid*, p. 4.
51. Edward Jenner, *An Inquiry into the Causes and Effects of . . . the Cow Pox* (1798), pp. 58-61.
52. *Ibid*, p. 60.
53. Angelo Gatti, *New Observations on Inoculation* (1768), pp. 8, 9.
54. Lady Montagu, *op. cit.*
55. James Burges, *An Account of the Preparation and Management Necessary to Inoculation* (1764), pp. 2, 8, 14.
56. *Ibid*, p. 11.
57. Mitland, *op. cit.*, pp. 26-28.
58. James Moore, *History of Smallpox and Vaccination* (1815), p. 254.
59. Rogers, *op. cit.*, p. 178.
60. Thomas Dudley Fosbroke, *Berkeley Manuscripts* (1821), p. 221.
61. Alexander Monro, *An Account of the Inoculation of the Small Pox in Scotland* (1765), p. 488.
62. William Woodville, *The History of the Inoculation of the Small-Pox in Great Britain* (1796), pp. 347, 348.
63. Charles Creighton, *The History of Epidemics*, Vol. 2 (1896), p. 513.
64. George Baker, *An Enquiry into the Merits of a Method of Inoculating the Small-Pox, which is now practised in several Counties of England* (1766), pp. 57, 59, 64, 65.
65. *The Northampton Mercury*, 15th December, 1768.
66. See *The British Medical Journal*, XI (1910), pp. 633-34.
67. Woodville, *op. cit.*, pp. 347, 348.
68. John Andrew, *The Practice of Inoculation Impartially Considered* (1765), p. 10.
69. Dimsdale, *op. cit.*, p. 82.
70. Giles Watts, *A Vindication of the New Method of Inoculating the Small-Pox* (1767), pp. 47, 48.
71. *The Gentleman's Magazine*, XLIX (1779), p. 247.
72. *The Gentleman's Magazine*, LVIII (1788), I, p. 283.
73. Daniel Sutton, *op. cit.*, p. 91.

74. William Woodville, *Advice to Parents on . . . Small-Pox* (1797), pp. 32, 33.
75. W. A. Greenhill, "Registers of Hastings Parishes", *Sussex Archaeological Collections*, XIV (1862), p. 200.
76. Heslop, *op. cit.*, p. 6.
77. Newman, *op. cit.*, p. 34.
78. "A List of the Persons Inoculated with the Small Pox by Robert Waller, Apothecary in Gosport in the Years 1722 and 1723", *Inoculation Letters, op. cit.*, p. 67.
79. "A Letter from Claudius Amyand Esqr., Dated Febry 6th 1725", *Inoculation Letters, op. cit.*, pp. 193-197.
80. Watts, *op. cit.*, pp. iv, v.
81. Dimsdale, *op. cit.*, pp. 1, 2, 78.
82. William Watson, *An Account of a Series of Experiments . . . of Inoculating the Small-Pox* (1768), p. 7.
83. *Ibid*, pp. 6-18.
84. Sutton, *op. cit.*, p. 77.
85. Watson, *op. cit.*, pp. 6-18.
86. Heslop, *op. cit.*, p. 9.
87. The evidence for this statement will be found in later sections of the book.
88. J. G. Scheuchzer, *An Account of the Success of Inoculating the Small-Pox* (1729), p. 24.
89. Jurin, *op. cit.*, p. 215.
90. *Ibid*.
91. Robert J. Thornton, *Facts Decisive in Favour of the Cow-Pock* (1803), p. 55.
92. *The Gentleman's Magazine*, 58 (1788), No. 1, p. 283.
93. Monro, *op. cit.*, p. 488.
94. Allan W. Downie, "Smallpox" in Stuart Mudd (Ed), *Infectious Agents and Host Reactions* (1970), p. 489.
95. Andrew, *op. cit.*, p. 15.
96. Dimsdale, *op. cit.*, p. 1.
97. *Ibid*, p. 2.
98. *Ibid*.
99. Barnes, *op. cit.*, p. 22.
100. Dixon, *op. cit.*, p. 243.
101. Houlton, *A Sermon, op. cit.*, p. 41.
102. Jenner, *An Inquiry, op. cit.*, pp. 58-61.
103. Watts, *op. cit.*, p. v.
104. James Hallifax, "An Authentic Account of the State of Inoculation at Ewell, in Surry", *Gentleman's Magazine* (1766), pp. 413, 414.
105. *The Northampton Mercury*, February 16th, 1778.
106. George Pearson, *An Inquiry Concerning the History of the Cow Pox* (1798), p. 79.
107. *Royal Commission on Vaccination*, 3rd Report (1890).

108. Sir John Sinclair, *The Statistical Account of Scotland*, 2 (1792), pp. 569-71.

109. Dr J Forbes, "Some Account of the Small-Pox lately prevalent in Chichester and its Vicinity", *London Medical Repository*, XVIII (1822), pp. 213, 219, 220.

110. *Ibid.*

111. C. D. Rosenwald, "Variolation and other observations made during a Smallpox Epidemic in the Southern Province of Tanganika", *The Medical Officer*, March 1951, p. 88.

112. P. J. Imperato, "The Practice of Variolation among the Songhai of Mali", *Transactions of the Royal Society of Tropical Medicine and Hygiene*, 62 (1968), p. 871; P. J. Imperato, "Observations on Variolation Practice in Mali", *Tropical and Geographical Medicine*, 26 (1974), p. 435.

113. N. May, *Impartial Remarks on the Suttonian Method* (1770), p. 152.

114. P. J. Imperato, *Observations, op. cit.*, p. 433.

115. *Ibid*, p. 432.

116. Maitland, *op. cit.*, p. 27.

117. Holwell, *op. cit.*, pp. 3, 4.

118. May, *op. cit.*, p. 152.

119. Dixon, *op. cit.*

120. *Ibid.*

121. J. Watkinson, *An Examination of a Charge brought against Inoculation* (1777), p. 17.

122. J. C. Lettsom, *A Letter . . . upon General Inoculation* (1778), p. 11; J. C. Lettsom, *Observations on Baron Dimsdale's Remarks on Dr Lettsom's "Letter . . . etc."*, p. 24.

123. T. Dimsdale, *Observations on the Introduction to the Plan of the Dispensary for General Inoculation* (1778), pp. 39-44.

124. Quoted in Lettsom, *Observations . . .* , pp. 19, 20.

125. J. Haygarth, *An Inquiry how to Prevent the Small-Pox* (Chester 1785), p. 188.

126. See P. E. Razzell, "Edward Jenner: The History of a Medical Myth", *Medical History*, X, No. 3 (July 1965), p. 216.

127. J. Haygarth, *A Sketch of a Plan to Exterminate the Casual Small-Pox* (1793), pp. 82, 83.

128. *Ibid*, pp. 78, 79.

129. Dixon, *op. cit.*, p. 297.

130. Haygarth, *A Sketch, op. cit.*, pp. 472-475.

131. William Woodville, *Reports of a Series of Inoculations for the Variolae Vaccine or Cowpox* (1799), pp. 151-155.

132. Haygarth, *A Sketch, op. cit.*, p. 129.

133. Quoted in William Woodville, *The History of the Inoculation of the Smallpox in Great Britain* (1796), p. 226.

134. See *The Royal Commission on Vaccination*, 4th Report (1893), p. 21.

135. John Mudge, *A Dissertation on the Inoculated Smallpox* (1777), p. 16.

136. William Woodville, *Advice to Parents on . . . Small Pox and . . . Inoculation . . .* (1797), p. 18.

137. S. S. Marennikova and R. A. Shafikova, "Comparative Studies on the Properties of Variola Virus Strains", *Acta Virologica*, 13 (1969).

138. R. A. Shafikova and S. S. Marennikova, "Characteristics of Properties of Variola Virus Strains Isolated from Patients with different forms of the Disease", *Voprosy Virusol*, 15 (1970).

139. K. R. Dumbell and Farida Huq, "Epidemiological Implications of the Typing of Variola Isolates", *Transactions of the Royal Society of Tropical Medicine and Hygiene*, 69 (1975), p. 306.

140. J. K. Sarkar *et. al.*, "Virus Excretion in Smallpox", *Bulletin of the World Health Organisation*, 48 (1973), p. 521.

141. Dixon, *op. cit.*, p. 298.

142. W. W. Peter, *The Heavenly Flower: Small Pox* (Undated), p. 15.

143. See Joseph Needham, *The Grand Titration* (1969), p. 59; C. A. Gordon, *An Epitome of the Reports to the Chinese Imperial Maritime Customs Service* (1884), pp. 78-81. The Chinese method of inoculation was tried on a seventh female convict in the Newgate Prison experiment of 1721, and although her inoculation was eventually as successful as that of the others in terms of the number of pustules, etc., she was "miserably tormented with sharp pains in her head, and a fever, which never left her till the eruption of the pustules". See Richard Mead, M.D., *A Discourse on the Small-Pox* (1748), p. 89.

144. Gordon, *op. cit.*, p. 79.

145. E. Frederick Wheelock, "Interferon in Dermal Crusts of Human Vaccinia Virus Vaccinations possible explanation of relative benignity of Variolation Smallpox", *Proceedings of the Society for Experimental Biology and Medicine*, 117 (1964).

146. Daniel Sutton, *op. cit.*, pp. 16, 17.

147. *Ibid.*

148. A. B. Christie, "Smallpox", *Infectious Diseases* (1974), pp. 210, 217.

149. Downie, *op. cit.*, p. 504.

150. H. S. Bedson, *The Ceiling Temperature of Pox Viruses* (University of London, M.B. Thesis, 1964).

151. A Kirn et J. Braunwald, "Selection par Passages a Basse Témperature d'un Variant 'Froid' a Virulence Atténuée du Virus Vaccinal", *Annales de l'Institut Pasteur*, 106 (1964), p. 438.

152. Derrick Baxby, "A possible relation between Human Pato-
     genicity of Smallpox Vaccines and Virus growth at elevated
     temperatures", *Journal of Hygiene, Cambridge,* 73 (1974),
     p. 35.
153. K. R. Dumbell, H. S. Bedson and Md. Nizamuddin, "Thermo-
     Efficient Strains of Variola Major Virus", *Journal of General
     Virology,* I (1967), pp. 379-381.
154. J. C. G. Leddingham and D. McClean, *British Journal of
     Experimental Pathology,* Vol. 9 (1928), pp. 218-224.
155. J. G. Scheuchzer, *An Account of the Success of Inoculating
     the Small-Pox* (1729), p. 24.
156. Creighton, *op. cit.,* p. 504.
157. Miller, *op. cit.,* p. 137.
158. *Ibid,* p. 132.
159. *Ibid,* p. 133.
160. C. Deering, *An Account of an improved Method of treating
     the Small-Pocks* (Nottingham 1737), p. 29.
161. S. H. A. Hervey (ed.), "The Diary of John Hervey, First Earl
     of Bristol, 1688-1742", *Suffolk Green Books,* II (1894), p. 84.
162. Dixon, *op. cit.,* p. 236.
163. Miller, *op. cit.,* p. 133.
164. *British Medical Journal* (1948), Vol. I, p. 79.
165. *Bristol Infirmary, Biographical Memoirs,* I, p. 60.
166. *The Gentleman's Magazine,* XX (1750), p. 532.
167. *Ibid,* XXII (1752), pp. 511-513.
168. Robert Cowie, M.D., *Shetland: Descriptive and Historical*
     (1871), pp. 73-75.
169. *Inoculation Letters, op. cit.*
170. Miller, *op. cit.,* pp. 3-7.
171. Andrew, *op. cit.,* p. 24.
172. *Ibid,* p. x.
173. E. M. Crookshank, *History and Pathology of Vaccination,*
     Vol. I (1889), p. 44.
174. *Dodsley's Annual Register,* XI (1768), p. 93.
175. W. Andrews (Ed.), *The Doctor: In History, Literature and
     Folklore* (1896), pp. 156-7.
176. D. Hartley, *Some Reasons why the Practice of Inoculation
     ought to be introduced into the Town of Bury at Present*
     (1733), pp. 7-15.
177. *Ibid.*
178. Miller, *op. cit.,* p. 169.
179. Houlton, *A Sermon, op. cit.,* p. 24.
180. Heslop, *op. cit.,* pp. 7, 8.
181. *The Northampton Mercury,* 7th September 1788.
182. W. Turner, *An Address to Parents on Inoculation for the
     Small-Pox* (Newcastle 1792), p. 10.
183. I. E. Gray (ed.), *Gloucester Quarter Session Archives 1660-
     1889* (Gloucester 1958), p. 17.

184. S. and B. Webb, *English Local Government—English Poor Law History* (1927), I, p. 306.
185. Heslop, *op. cit.*, p. 9.
186. *Ibid*, 10.
187. R. Hine, *The History of Beaminster* (Taunton 1914), pp. 429, 430.
188. W. Holloway, *The History of Rye* (1847), p. 440.
189. See for example F. W. Steer, "A Relic of an Eighteenth Century Isolation Hospital", *The Lancet*, CCLXX (1956), pp. 200, 201; E. G. Erith, *Essex Parish Records, 1240-1894* (1950), p. 25; E. G. Thomas, *The Parish Overseer in Essex, 1597-1834* (London M.A. Thesis 1956).
190. Thomas, *op. cit.*, p. 394.
191. "Letter from Rev. Mr. Stuart", *Gentleman's Magazine*, 58, No. I (1788), p. 284.
192. *Ibid*.
193. Thomas, *op. cit.*, pp. 164, 165.
194. Thomas Dimsdale, *Thoughts on General and Partial Inoculations* (1776), p. 29.
195. *Ibid*, pp. 62, 63.
196. John Baron, *The Life of Edward Jenner*, Vol. I (1838), p. 434.
197. G. P. Scrope, *History of Castle Combe* (1852), pp. 383, 384.
198. Dimsdale, *Thoughts, op. cit.*, p. 63.
199. Thomas Glass, M.D., *A Letter . . . to Dr Baker on . . . Small Pox* (1767), p. 55.
200. Watson, *op. cit.*, pp. 71, 72.
201. W. Buchan, *Domestic Medicine* (1769), p. 237.
202. H. W. Carter, "General Report of Medical Diseases treated at the Kent and Canterbury Hospital, 1824", *London Medical Repository*, XXII (1824), p. 268.
203. John Cross, *A History of the Variolous Epidemic which occurred in Norwich* (1820), p. 272.
204. *The Gentleman's Magazine*, XXIII (1753), p. 217.
205. *Ibid*.
206. Buchan, *op. cit.*, pp. 233, 234.
207. R. L. Hine, *The History of Hitchin*, 2 (1929), pp. 117, 118.
208. Turner, *op. cit.*, p. 10.
209. *Medical Commentaries*, 2nd Decade, I (1786), pp 244, 245.
210. Thomas Alston Warren, *An Address from a Country Minister to his Parishioners on the Subject of the Cow-Pox* (1803), p. 9.
211. Haygarth, *A Sketch of a Plan, op. cit.*, p. 186.
212. *Ibid*.
213. *The Gentleman's Magazine*, 49 (1779), p. 193.
214. Baker, *op. cit.*, pp. 64, 65.
215. Dimsdale, *Thoughts, op. cit.*, pp. 32, 33.
216. Haygarth, *A Sketch, op. cit.*, p. 482.

217. John Franks, "Letter from John Franks, Smith Street, Westminster, November 7, 1800", *Medical and Physical Journal*, 4 (1800), p. 519.
218. *The Monthly Ledger*, I (1775), p. 523.
219. Miller, *op. cit.*, p. 169.
220. *Ibid.*
221. *Ibid*, p. 170.
222. Hine, *The History of Beaminster, op. cit.*, pp. 429, 430.
223. Webbs, *op. cit.*, p. 306, fn. 2.
224. Moore, *op. cit.*, p. 247.
225. See Miller, *op. cit.*, p. 137.
226. Dixon, *op. cit.*, p. 239.
227. *The Gentleman's Magazine*, XX (1750), p. 532.
228. *Ibid*, XXIII (1753), p. 217.
229. J. Kirkpatrick, *The Analysis of Inoculation* (1754), pp. 267, 268.
230. *The Gentleman's Magazine*, XXI (1751), p. 152.
231. *Ibid*, XXII (1752), pp. 511-513.
232. W. H. Jones, *Bradford-On-Avon* (1907), p. 64.
233. Woodville, *History of Inoculation, op. cit.*, pp. 221, 222; Dixon, *op. cit.*, p. 197.
234. Creighton, *op. cit.*, p. 513.
235. Gray, *op. cit.*, p. 17.
236. W. Holloway, *The History of Rye* (1847), p. 440.
237. Creighton, *op. cit.*, p. 504.
238. The basis of this estimate is unknown to me, but it is probable that it was more or less a guess made in connection with an inquiry conducted under the auspices of the French Government. For the estimate, see A. C. Klebs, "The Historic Evolution of Variolation", *Bulletin of the Johns Hopkins Hospital*, XXIV (1913), p. 82.
239. Andrew, *op. cit.*, pp. 5, 65.
240. *The Monthly Ledger*, I (1775), pp. 522-527.
241. *Ibid*, p. 524.
242. Woodville, *History of Inoculation, op. cit.*, pp. 345, 346.
243. Baker, *op. cit.*, pp. 64, 65.
244. *Royal Commission on Vaccination*, 3rd Report (1890), p. 53.
245. *Considerations on the Dearness of Corn and Provisions* [Author Anonymous] (1767), p. 7.
246. Edmonston, *op. cit.*, p. 87.
247. *Ibid.*
248. "Letters from Mr Thomas Davies to Mr Hodgson", *Glynde Estate Archives* (East Sussex Record Office, MSS 2772).
249. Houlton, *A Sermon, op. cit.*, p. 47.
250. Houlton, *The Tryal, op. cit.*, p. 6.
251. Daniel Sutton, *op. cit.*, p. 60.
252. Woodville, *History of Inoculation, op. cit.*, p. 350.
253. Daniel Sutton, *op. cit.*, p. viii.

254. Robert Houlton, *Indisputable Facts Relative to the Suttonian Art of Inoculation* (Dublin 1768), p. 20.

255. *Ibid*, pp. 21-23.

256. *The Gentleman's Magazine*, LXVI, i (1796), p. 112.

257. G. Lipscomb, *A Manual of Inoculation* (1806), p. 30.

258. Woodville, *History of Inoculation, op. cit.*, p. 350.

259. Daniel Sutton, *op. cit.*, p. xiii.

260. J. J. Abraham, *Lettsom* (1933), p. 195, fn. 2.

261. Dixon, *op. cit.*, p. 243.

262. Dorothy Fisk, *Doctor Jenner of Berkeley* (1959), p. 117.

263. Dixon, *op. cit.*, p. 244.

264. Quoted in May, *op. cit.*, pp. 176-178.

265. *Gorton's Biographical Dictionary*, Vol. 2, p. 975.

266. G. Pearson, *An Inquiry Concerning the History of the Cowpox* (1798), p. 102.

267. Heslop, *op. cit.*, pp. 7, 8.

268. Houlton, *Indisputable Facts, op. cit.*, p. 41.

269. J. Howlett, *Observations on the Increased Population . . . Of Maidstone* (Maidstone, 1782), p. 8.

270. The Webbs, *op. cit.*, p. 306, fn. 2. See also Thomas, *op. cit.*, p. 169, and M. F. Davies, *Life in an English Village* (1909), p. 74, for further references to compulsory inoculation.

271. R. Hine, *The History of Beaminster* (Taunton 1914), pp. 429, 430.

272. *Ibid.*

273. Jenner, *Inquiry, op. cit.*, in Crookshank, *op. cit.*, Vol. 2, p. 30.

274. Edward Jenner, "On the Origin of the Vaccine Inoculation" (1801) in Crookshank, *op. cit.*, Vol. 2, p. 271.

275. Jenner, *Inquiry, op. cit.*, in Crookshank, *op. cit.*, Vol. 2, p. 30.

276. J. Watkinson, *An Examination of a Charge Brought Against Inoculation* (1777), p. 28.

277. W. Black, *Observations Medical and Political on the Small Pox and Inoculation* (1781), Appendix, p. 2.

278. J. Aikin, "The Bill of Mortality of the Town of Warrington, for the year 1773", *Philosophical Transactions*, 64 (1774), p. 440.

279. T. Percival, "Observations on the State of Population in Manchester and other Adjacent Places", in the author's *Essays Medical, Philosophical, and Experimental*, Vol. 2 (1776), pp. 6, 7.

280. J. Haygarth, *An Inquiry, op. cit.*, p. 164.

281. See Creighton, *op. cit.*, pp. 505, 506, for a discussion of the London Smallpox Hospital.

282. J. C. Lettsom, *A Letter to Sir Robert Baker and George Stacpoole Esq. Upon General Inoculation* (1778), p. 43.

283. *Ibid.*

284. See Creighton, *op. cit.*, p. 507, for a summary of these events.

285. It is possible that free inoculation was practised after 1794 by a General Dispensary planned in that year. See the *Plan of the General Dispensary for Inoculating and Administering Advice and Medicines Gratis to all the Infant Poor, at their own Habitations, and at the Dispensary, Wardour Street, Soho, Three Doors from Oxford Street* (1794).

286. G. Gregory, *Some Account of the Hospital for Small-Pox and Vaccination* (1830).

287. Watkinson, *op. cit.*, p. 28.

288. *The Gentleman's Magazine*, LXXIII, ii (1803), p. 71.

289. *Royal Commission Report on Vaccination*, 6th Report (1896), p. 360.

290. Joseph Adams, *An Inquiry into the Laws of Epidemics* (1809), p. 143.

291. Creighton, *op. cit.*, pp. 589, 590.

292. *The London Medical Repository*, 4 (1815), p. 174.

293. Haygarth, *A Sketch, op. cit.*, p. 127.

294. See Creighton, *op. cit.*, pp. 510, 511, for a summary of this evidence.

295. *The Gentleman's Magazine*, LX, ii (1790), p. 732.

296. *ibid*, pp. 511, 512.

297. Haygarth, *A Sketch, op. cit.*, p. 482.

293. *Report of The Royal College of Physicians of London on Vaccination* (1807), p. 6.

299. Creighton, *op. cit.*, p. 508.

300. *Ibid*.

301. *Ibid*.

302. *Ibid*.

303. *Ibid*, p. 511. It must not be assumed that because only a minority of the population was at risk, that the population was of less need of protection (as Creighton implied); it was simply that smallpox was virtually endemic in Chester and therefore the population at risk were infants and young children who are bound to be a minority of the total population at any one point of time.

304. Haygarth, *A Sketch, op. cit.*, p. 186.

305. J. Heysham, "An Abridgement of the Observations on the Bills of Mortality in Carlisle, from the year 1779 to 1787, inclusive", published in W. Hutchinson, *The History of Cumberland* (1794), pp. 668-75. Professor Glass has stated that "the claims made by Heysham do not appear to tally with the numbers he himself reports as having been inoculated at the city dispensary" [Glass and Eversley, *op. cit.*, p. 18, fn. 73], but it is difficult to know what the basis of this criticism is. The only year where it is possible to check Heysham's claims against the original bills is 1786/7, in which Heysham claimed that "eighty-four were inoculated at the

dispensary", an identical number to that stated in the original bill as having been inoculated at the dispensary.

306. R. Walker, *An Inquiry into the Small-Pox* (1790), p. 467, fn.

307. *Report of the Royal College of Physicians, op. cit.* This report is to be found in the Royal College of Physicians' library in London, along with all the original evidence (letters sent to the College) which is arranged by numbers. In quoting this evidence I shall cite *"Evidence to Royal College of Physicians,* Letter No. etc."

308. *Evidence to The Royal College of Physicians,* Letter No. 132.

309. *Ibid,* Letter No. 150. See also Creighton, *op. cit.,* pp. 582-584, for confirmation of this point.

310. *Letter from Dr Walker to Dr Lettsom, Oct. 9th 1801* (Wellcome Institute for the History of Medicine Library, Letter No. 16486).

311. J. Birch, *Tracts on Vaccination* (1817), p. 24.

312. *Letter No. 5, Jenner's Letters,* in Royal College of Physicians' Library.

313. John Conolly, *Observations on Vaccinations and on the Practice of Inoculating for the Small-Pox* (Stratford-On-Avon, 1824), p. 67.

314. *MSS D/P 70/12/3* (Berkshire Record Office).

315. Conolly, *op. cit.,* p. 68.

316. John Cross, *A History of the Variolous Epidemic which occurred in Norwich* (1820), pp. 13, 219.

317. *Ibid,* p. 219.

318. *Ibid,* p. 220.

319. J. Forbes, "Some Account of the Small-Pox Lately Prevalent in Chichester and its Vicinity", *London Medical Repository,* 18 (1822), pp. 211, 212.

320. *Ibid,* p. 213.

321. See Creighton, *op. cit.,* pp. 582-85, for a discussion of the spread of vaccination in these places.

322. See B. R. Mitchell and P. Deane, *Abstract of British Historical Statistics* (Cambridge 1962), pp. 8, 24-27.

323. W. Rowley, *Cow-Pox Inoculation no Security Against Small-Pox Infection* (1805), p. 4.

324. *Parliamentary Debates (Hansard),* 3rd Series, Vol. 52, Feb.-March 1840, p. 1195.

325. Thomas Dimsdale, *Thoughts on General and Partial Inoculations* (1776), pp. 32, 33.

326. Thomas Dimsdale, *Observations on the Introduction to the Plan of the Dispensary for General Inoculation* (1778), pp. 58, 59. See also *The Monthly Review,* 58 (1778), pp. 297, 298.

327. *The Monthly Review,* 58 (1778), pp. 297, 298.

328. Thomas Dimsdale, *Tracts on Inoculation* (1781), pp. 104, 105.

329. Dimsdale, *Thoughts, op. cit.,* pp. 31-33.

330. Dimsdale, *Observations, op. cit.,* p. 126.

174

331. J. Haygarth, *An Inquiry, op. cit.*, p. 164.
332. Howlett, *op. cit.*, p. 8.
333. I am grateful to E. G. Thomas for supplying these references to me. The main source is *All Saints and St. Peter's Register, Maldon*, although the inoculation for 1764 is that previously discussed in connection with Daniel Sutton, and the reference to the 1779 inoculation is taken from *The Gentleman's Magazine*, IL (1779), p. 193.
334. Edward Jenner, *Further Observations on the Variolae Vaccinae* (1799), in Crookshank, *op. cit.*, Vol. 2, p. 164.
335. Jenner, *Inquiry, op. cit.*, in Crookshank, *op. cit.*, Vol. 2, p. 10.
336. *Ibid*, p. 17.
337. G. C. Jenner, "An Account of a General Inoculation at Painswick", *The London Medical Journal*, Vol. 7 (1786), p. 163.
338. *Ibid*.
339. Heslop, *op. cit.*, pp. 9, 10.
340. *Ibid*, p. 10.
341. "The Small Pox and General Inoculations", *Town Book of Lewes, 1702-1837*, pp. 94-96.
342. *Ipswich Journal*, 6th June 1784.
343. *Ipswich Journal*, 20th June 1778.
344. W. A. Barron, "Gleanings From Sussex Archives: Brighton and the Smallpox", *The Sussex County Magazine*, 26 (1952), pp. 605, 606.
345. C. Wright, *The Brighton Ambulator* (1818), p. 102.
346. "Notes on Occurrences", *Tenterden Parish Register* (Kent County Archive Office).
347. Jenner, *Further Observations, op. cit.*, in Crookshank, *op. cit.*, Vol. 2, p. 182.
348. See T. Beddoes, "Queries Respecting a Safer Method of Performing Inoculation" in Don A. De Gimbernat (Beddoes translator), *A New Method for the General Hernia* (1795), pp. 56-59.
349. J. Blake, *Public Health in the Town of Boston, 1630-1822* (Cambridge, U.S.A., 1959), p. 244; *Royal Commission on Vaccination*, 6th Report (1896), p. 762; H. R. Viets (ed.), *A Brief Rule to Guide the Common People of New England* (Baltimore, 1937), p. 35.
350. Blake, *op. cit.*
351. *Ibid*.
352. Alexander Monro, "Account of the Inoculation of Small-Pox in Scotland (1765)", in A. Monro, *The Works of Alexander Monro, M.D.* (Edinburgh 1781), p. 693.
353. *Ibid*, p. 682.
354. A. Aberdour, *Observations on the Smallpox and Inoculation* (Edinburgh 1791), p. 61.
355. See Sir J. Sinclair (Ed.), *The Statistical Account of Scotland*, 21 vols. (Edinburgh 1791-99).

356. *Ibid*, Vol. 4 (1792), p. 133.
357. *Ibid*, Vol. 2 (1792), p. 119.
358. *Ibid*, Vol. 20 (1798), pp. 143, 144.
359. *Ibid*, Vol. 2 (1792), p. 119.
360. Monro, *op. cit.*, p. 680.
361. *Ibid*.
362. Sinclair, *op. cit.*, Vol. 2 (1792), pp. 452, 453.
363. *Ibid*, Vol. 7 (1794), p. 320.
364. *Evidence to The Royal College of Physicians, op. cit.*, Letter No. 30.
365. Houlton, *Indisputable Facts, op. cit.*, p. 25.
366. See T. W. Freeman, *Pre-Famine Ireland* (Manchester 1957), p. 27.
367. In April 1777, "Agreeable to the humane resolutions of the King's County Infirmary, 461 persons were, in the course of last month, inoculated." See Population Census of Ireland 1851, *Parl. Pap. 1856/29*, p. 422.
368. Population Census of Ireland 1841, *Parl. Pap. 1843/24*, p. xii.
369. De Latocnaye (Translator John Stevenson), *A Frenchman's Walk Through Ireland 1796-97* (Dublin 1917), pp. 175-177.
370. James Moore, *The History and Practice of Vaccination (1817)*, p. 228.
371. "Report on Vaccination in Ireland by the Royal Dublin College of Physicians", appendix to the *Report of the Royal College of Physicians of London on Vaccination* (1807), p. 8.
372. *Evidence to Royal College of Physicians, op. cit.*, Letter No. 8.
373. "Report on Vaccination in Ireland . . . ", *op. cit.*, p. 8.
374. H. Townsend, *Statistical Survey of the County of Cork* (1810), p. 90.
375. *Evidence to Royal College of Physicians, op. cit.*, Letter No. 8.
376. *Ibid*.
377. See *The Epidemiological Society Report* (1852-53), p. 29.
378. Dimsdale, *Observations, op. cit.*, pp. 29, 30.
379. See K. C. Hurd-Mead, *A History of Women in Medicine* (1938), p. 505. According to Hurd-Mead inoculation was made compulsory by law in these three countries, although there is considerable doubt as to how effective these laws were.
380. See P. L. Logan, "The Inoculation of Smallpox—Dr Timotes O'Scanlan", *Journal of the Irish Medical Association*, 54 (1964), p. 56. In a book written by O'Scanlan (in about 1800?), he stated that only 31,000 people had been inoculated in Spain and Colonies since 1771.
381. Dixon, *op. cit.*, p. 5.
382. T. Dimsdale, *Tracts on Inoculation* (1781), pp. 176-78.
383. See for example *Surrey Archaeological Collections*, XXVII (1914), pp. 16-20, for a description and an enumeration of individual cases of people dying from smallpox during epidemics which occurred in Godalming, Surrey in 1672, 1686,

1701, 1710-11 and 1722-23. Contemporaries were much more familiar with smallpox than we are today and this would have enabled them to avoid confusing the disease with other diseases.

384. See *The London Bills of Mortality* in the Guildhall Library.
385. Dixon, *op. cit.*, pp. 4-12.
386. *Ibid*, p. 324.
387. See E. W. and A. E. Stearn, *The Effect of Smallpox on the Destiny of the Ameriandian* (Boston, 1945).
388. K. Dewhurst (Ed.), *Dr Thomas Sydenham, 1624-89* (1966), pp. 106, 119.
389. *The Gentleman's Magazine*, XLII (1772), p. 542.
390. G. Utterström, "Some population problems in pre-industrial Sweden", *Scandinavian Econ. Hist. Rev.*, 3 (1955), p. 131.
391. T. Short, *A History of the Air, Weather, Seasons, etc.* (1749), 1, p. 354.
392. T. Percival, *Arguments against the Inoculation of Children in Early Infancy* (Dublin 1768), p. 116. For other examples of contemporary comments on deaths from smallpox amongst young infants where death occurred before the eruption of pustules and was associated with convulsive fits, see Dr Mead, *A Treatise on the Small-Pox and Measles* (1747), pp. 40, 45; William Buchan, *Domestic Medicine* (Edinburgh 1769), pp. 253, 255; A. Aberdour, *Observations on the Small-Pox and Inoculation* (Edinburgh 1791), p. 76.
393. James Jurin, *An Account of the Success of Inoculating the Small-Pox* (1727), p. 22.
394. Monro, *op. cit.*, pp. 487, 690, 691.
395. See for example Creighton, *op. cit.*, p. 491, and *The Gentleman's Magazine*, LVIII, i (1788), p. 284.
396. Haygarth, *A Sketch, op. cit.*, p. 141.
397. *Royal Commission on Vaccination*, 6th Report (1896), p. 270.
398. *Medical Observations and Inquiries*, V (1776), p. 272.
399. *Philosophical Transactions*, LXVIII (1788), p. 150.
400. See *St. Giles Cripplegate (London) Burial Dues, 1774-93* and *St. Brides (London) Burial Register, 1736-1812*, both lodged in the Guildhall Library.
401. Dixon, *op. cit.*, p. 149.
402. *Surrey Archaeological Collections*, XXVII (1914), pp. 16-20.
403. Creighton, *op. cit.*, p. 534. See also Lettsom, *A Letter, op. cit.*, p. 5.
404. *Royal Commission on Vaccination*, 6th Report (1896), p. 265; Creighton, *op. cit.*, p. 749.
405. T. J. Pettigrew, *Memoirs of the Life and Writings of the Late John Coakley Lettsom* (1817), Vol. I, p. 41.
406. P. Newman, *Malaria Eradication and Population Growth* (University of Michigan, 1965), p. 10.

407. J. Jurin, *An Account of the Success of Inoculating the Small-Pox* (1724), pp. 27, 28.

408. J. C. Lettsom, *A Letter to Sir Robert Baker and George Stacpole Esq. Upon General Inoculation* (1778), pp. 5, 6.

409. Watts, *op. cit.*, p. 53.

410. Robert Willan, *Reports of the Diseases in London* (1800), p. 313.

411. *Surrey Archaeological Collections*, XVIII (1914), p. 20.

412. Dixon, *op. cit.*, p. 88.

413. W. T. Councilman *et. al.*, "The Pathological Anatomy and Histology of Variola", in *Studies on the Pathology and on the Etiology of Variola and of Vaccination* (1909), pp. 69, 70.

414. I am grateful to Professor Keith Dumbell for this information on the possible relationship between smallpox and tuberculosis.

415. Councilman, *op. cit.*

416. *Ibid*, p. 92.

417. G. Bras, "The Morbid Anatomy of Smallpox", *Documenta De Medicina Et Tropica*, 4 (1952), p. 341.

418. A. M. Phadke, *et. al.*, "Smallpox as an Etiologic Factor in Male Infertility", *Fertility and Sterility*, 24 (1973), pp. 802-804.

419. F. Bellinger, M.D., *A Treatise Concerning the Small-Pox* (1721), pp. 23, 24; George Pearson, Thornton, *op. cit.*, p. 54.

420. A. R. Rao, *et. al.*, "Pregnancy and Smallpox", *Journal of the Indian Medical Association*, 40 (1963), pp. 353-362.

421. *Bristol Infirmary, Biographical Memoirs*, I, p. 60.

422. Haygarth, *A Sketch, op. cit.*, p. 381.

423. Quoted in M. D. George, *London Life in the Eighteenth Century* (1925), p. 348, fn. 4.

424. J. Dunkin, *History of Dartford* (1844), p. 397.

425. Dimsdale, *Observations, op. cit.*, pp. 79, 80.

426. "Letter From Mr Thomas Chubbs, Sarum, 10th August, 1723", *Inoculation Letters, op. cit.*, p. 60.

427. *Maidstone Burial Register* (1760), in the Maidstone Parish Church.

428. R. L. Hine, *The History of Hitchin*, I (1927), pp. 265, 266 fn.

429. *Royal Commission on Vaccination*, 6th Report (1896), p. 262.

430. D. D'Escheruy, *An Essay on the Smallpox* (1760), p. 2.

431. Dixon, *op. cit.*, pp. 190, 191.

432. For the original information on which the above figures were compiled see *The Parish Register of Allhallows London Wall, 1559-1675* (Chiswick Press, 1878), in the Institute of Historical Research, London.

1846), p. 427.

433. John Stuart (Ed.), *Selections from the Records of the Kirk Session, Presbytry and Synod of Aberdeen*, 1 (Aberdeen,

434. *Parish Register of Holy Trinity, Chester, 1532-1837* (1914), p. 199.

435. *Royal Commission on Vaccination,* 6th Report (1896), p. 716.

436. See Creighton, *op. cit.,* p. 526.

437. G. Eland (Ed.), *Purefoy Letters, 1735-1753,* 2 (1931), p. 331.

438. See *MSS IC/992* and *MSS IC/1185* in the Northampton Record Office.

439. Edward J. Edwardes, M.D., *A Concise History of Smallpox and Vaccination in Europe* (1902), p. 13. Also see *Royal Commission on Vaccination,* 6th Report (1896), p. 268.

440. Hurd-Mead, *op. cit.*

441. W. J. Stavert (Ed.), *The Parish Register of Skipton-In-Craven* (Skipton, 1895).

442. *All Saints, Maidstone Parish Register.*

443. *Notes and Queries for Somerset and Dorset,* XX (1930-32), p. 124.

444. *Ibid.*

445. *Surrey Archaeological Collections,* XXVII (1914), pp. 16-20.

446. Creighton, *op. cit.,* p. 520.

447. *Inoculation Letters, op. cit.*

448. Creighton, *op. cit.,* p. 521.

449. "Riseley Parish Register", *Bedfordshire Parish Registers,* XXVIII, in the Bedfordshire Record Office.

450. *Bedfordshire Historical Record Society,* XVI (1934), p. 134.

451. Crookshank, *op. cit.,* Vol. I, p. 112.

452. *Royal Commission on Vaccination,* 1st Report (1889), pp. 109, 110.

453. R. Cowie, *Shetland: Descriptive and Historical* (Aberdeen, 1871), pp. 73-75; see also Sinclair, *Statistical Account of Scotland,* 20 (1798), p. 101, for another description of this epidemic.

454. Holwell, *op. cit.,* pp. 4, 5.

455. The Stearns, *op. cit.*

456. V. J. Derbes, "Smallpox in English Poetry of the Seventeenth Century", *American Med. Ass. Arch. Derm.,* 77 (1958), p. 430.

457. *MSS IC/845* in the Northamptonshire Record Office.

458. *Inoculation Letters, op. cit.,* p. 59.

459. Eland, *op. cit.,* p. 374.

460. Short, *A History, op. cit.,* pp. 411, 412.

461. *Ibid,* pp. 407, 408.

462. Jurin, *A Letter, op. cit.,* pp. 12, 13.

463. "A Letter From Mr Towgood to Dr Jurin, Shepton Mallet, Somerset, March 18, 1727", *Inoculation Letters, op. cit.,* p. 358.

464. James Jurin, *An Account of the Success of Inoculating the Small Pox* (1724), p. 17.

465. Gatti, *op. cit.,* p. 39.

466. Sloane, *op. cit.,* p. 519.

467. William Hillary, M.D., *A Practical Essay on the Small Pox* (1740), p. 32.
468. Bromfield, *op. cit.*, p. 16.
469. Thomas Thompson, *An Enquiry Into The Smallpox* (1752), pp. 1, 2.
470. *The Gentleman's Magazine,* IL (1779), p. 193.
471. W. Black, *Observations Medical and Political on the Smallpox and Inoculation* (1781), p. 68.
472. Haygarth, *A Sketch, op. cit.*, pp. 31, 32.
473. *Ibid,* p. 32.
474. T. J. Pettigrew, *Memoirs of the Life and Writings of the Late John Coakley Lettsom* (1817), 2, pp. 121, 122.
475. D. E. C. Eversley, "A Survey of Population in an Area of Worcestershire from 1660-1850 on the Basis of Parish Records", *Population Studies,* X (1956-57), p. 267.
476. According to a historian of Burford, "until the middle of the [eighteenth] century Burford was relying on its trade as a posting station . . . In 1761 a coach began running from Burford to London by way of Witney". R. H. Gretton, *The Burford Records* (Oxford, 1920), pp. 223, 224.
477. See the *Parish Register of Burford,* 1758. This register is lodged in the Bodleian Library, Oxford University.
478. James McKenzie, *The History of Health* (1760).
479. *Inoculation Letters, op. cit.*, p. 59.
480. *Ibid,* p. 92.
481. Nettleton, *op. cit.*, p. 51.
482. Haygarth, *A Sketch, op. cit.*, p. 31.
483. For the source of these figures, see Creighton, *op. cit.*, pp. 518, 519.
484. *Ibid,* p. 520.
485. *Royal Commission on Vaccination,* 6th Report (1896), p. 718.
486. W. Gayton, *The Value of Vaccination* (1885), p. 21.
487. J. C. McVail, *Half a Century of Small-Pox and Vaccination* (1919), p. 19.
488. The figures for 1574-98 are derived from the *Parish Register of Allhallows London Wall*; the rest from the *London Bills of Mortality*—see "Report on the State of Small-Pox and Vaccination in England and Wales and Other Countries . . . presented to the Epidemiological Society", *Parl. Pap. 1852-53/XLV,* p. 24, and Creighton, *op. cit.*, p. 436.
489. Creighton, *op. cit.*, p. 436.
490. See Miller, *op. cit.*, p. 30.
491. Dixon, *op. cit.*, p. 193.
492. *Surrey Archaeological Collections,* XXVII (1914), pp. 16-20; Stavert, *op. cit.*
493. Creighton, *op. cit.*, p. 519.
494. C. Deering, *Nottinghamia Vetus Et Nova* (Nottingham, 1751), p. 82.

495. Creighton, *op. cit.*, p. 519.
496. *Ibid*, p. 519, fn. 1.
497. W. Clinch, *An Historical Essay on the Rise and Progress of the Small-Pox* (1725), p. 40.
498. Short, *A History, op. cit.*, pp. 407, 408.
499. *Ibid*, pp. 518, 519.
500. "A Letter From Dr Nettleton to Dr Jurin, Halifax, November 11th 1723", *Inoculation Letters, op. cit.*, pp. 119-123.
501. Rev David Some, *The Case of Receiving the Small-Pox by Inoculation* (1750), p. 29.
502. Isaac Massey, *A Letter to the Learned James Jurin, M.D.* (1723), p. 10.
503. Some, *op. cit.*, p. 28.
504. Dixon, *op. cit.*, p. 326.
505. See *Royal Commission on Vaccination*, 1st Report (1889), p. 74, 3rd Report (1890), p. 100, 6th Report (1896), p. 717; *The Lancet*, 9 (Feb. 11, 1826), pp. 670, 671.
506. This was true as late as 1826-44. See the *Register Book of Patients Under Casual Smallpox at Small-Pox Hospital St. Pancras From 1st January 1827* in the Greater London Council library.
507. *Royal Commission on Vaccination*, 6th Report (1896), p. 717.
508. *Northampton Bills of Mortality* (1740).
509. *Ibid* (1747).
510. Dixon, *op. cit.*, p. 197.
511. *The Gentleman's Magazine*, 23 (1753), p. 218.
512. Creighton, *op. cit.*, p. 544.
513. *The London Medical Journal*, X (1789), p. 270 fn.
514. Percival, *op. cit.*, Appendix, p. 67.
515. *Royal Commission on Vaccination*, 1st Report (1889), p. 3.
516. *Royal Commission on Vaccination*, 2nd Report (1890), p. 39.
517. Edwardes, *op. cit.*, p. 105.
518. *Ibid*.
519. *Ibid*.
520. *Ibid*, p. 106.
521. *Ibid*.
522. Creighton, *op. cit.*, p. 520; F. W. Barry, M.D., *Report on an Epidemic of Small-Pox at Sheffield* (1889), p. 174.
523. See P. E. Razzell, "An Interpretation of the Modern Rise of Population in Europe—A Critique", *Population Studies*, 28 (1974).
524. Pettigrew, *op. cit.*, pp. 121, 122.
525. J. Fleetwood, *History of Medicine in Ireland* (Dublin, 1951), p. 65.
526. See Dr J. Rutty, *A Chronological History of the Weather and Seasons, and of the Prevailing Diseases in Dublin* (Dublin, 1770).
527. *Royal Commission on Vaccination*, 6th Report (1896), p. 284.

528. See J. Marshall, *Mortality of the Metropolis* (1832).

529. *Report of the Vaccine Pock Institution, 1800-02* (1803), p. 100; also Creighton, *op. cit.*, pp. 525, 540.

530. See *Maidstone Parish Register*.

531. T. Percival, *Essays, Medical, Philosophical and Experimental* (Warrington, 1785-9), 4th ed., p. 69.

532. Haygarth, *A Sketch, op. cit.*, p. 140.

533. *Ibid*, p. 141; J. Haygarth, "Observations on the Population and Diseases of Chester, in the year 1774", *Philosophical Transactions*, 68, No. 1 (1778), p. 152.

534. J. Howlett, *An Examination of Dr Price's Essay* (Maidstone, 1781), p. 83 fn.

535. Haygarth, *An Inquiry, op. cit.*, pp. 112, 113. See also the Lympsfield, Surrey parish register for an example of a few deaths from smallpox every two years or so during the period 1676 and 1752.

536. See the *Bray Monument* in Great Barrington parish church.

537. *Ibid*.

538. R. Pickard, *Population and Epidemics of Exeter* (1947), pp. 65, 66.

539. *Dodsley's Annual Register*, 5 (1762), p. 118.

540. Heslop, *op. cit.*, p. 10.

541. *Ibid*.

542. *Hungerford Vestry Book, 1794* (MSS D/P 71/8/1 in the Berkshire Record Office).

543. Dimsdale, *Observations, op. cit.*, pp. 58, 59; *The Monthly Review*, 58 (1778), pp. 297-98.

544. Dimsdale, *Observations, op. cit.*, p. 126.

545. Beddoes, *op. cit.*, pp. 56-59.

546. J. Blake, *Public Health in the Town of Boston, 1630-1822* (Cambridge, U.S.A., 1959), p. 244; *Royal Commission on Vaccination*, 6th Report (1896), p. 762; H. R. Viets (Ed.), *A Brief Rule to Guide the Common People of New England* (Baltimore, 1937), p. 35. The figures in this table do not balance, as some people inoculated were not inhabitants of the town, and were therefore not included in the total population.

547. Forbes, *op. cit.*, p. 215.

548. For the source of these statistics see *Maidstone All Saints Parish Register* lodged in the Church. After 1753 smallpox deaths are individually registered, but before this date the register simply states "small-pox now in this town" during epidemic years—thus the number of smallpox deaths for the period 1740-51 is an estimate based on changes in the total number of burials during epidemic years. The increase in the total number of burials during the whole period is a function of increasing population, e.g. the population was 5755 in 1782 and 8027 in 1801.

549. See the *Calne Parish Register* in the Wiltshire Archaeological Society Library at Devizes.

550. See the *Basingstoke Parish Register* lodged in the Genealogical Society Library for the source of the statistics quoted in the following discussion.

551. See the *Report of the Vaccine Pock Institution, 1800-02* (London, 1803), pp. 100, 101.

552. Haygarth, *A Sketch, op. cit.*, p. 141; J. Haygarth, "Observations on the Population and Diseases of 'Chester, in the Year 1774", *Philosophical Transactions*, 68, i (1778), p. 152.

553. *Holy Trinity Chester Parish Register.*

554. Haygarth, *A Sketch, op. cit.*, p. 186.

555. *Ibid*, p. 36.

556. Haygarth, *An Inquiry, op. cit.*, pp. 197, 201.

557. Haygarth, *A Sketch, op. cit.*, pp. 33, 34.

558. *Ibid.*, p. 34.

559. "Letter From Thomas Davies, 18 March 1767", *op. cit.*

560. See P. E. Razzell, "The Evaluation of Baptism as a Form of Birth Registration Through Cross-Matching Census and Parish Register Data", *Population Studies*, xxvi, No. 1 (March, 1972), p. 131.

561. George Gregory, *Lectures on the Eruptive Fevers* (1843), p. 94.

562. These statistics are compiled from the London Bills of Mortality. For the original statistics see J. Marshall, *Mortality of the Metropolis* (1832).

563. Dimsdale, *Thoughts, op. cit.*, pp. 32, 33.

564. C. F. Palmer, *The History of Tamworth* (Tamworth, 1845), p. 198.

565. The *Milton Ernest Parish Register*, lodged in the Genealogical Society Library (London).

566. See the *Horton Kirbie Parish Register*, lodged in the Genealogical Society Library.

567. See the *Whittington Parish Register*, lodged in the Genealogical Society Library.

568. For the statistics of Selattyn see the *Selattyn Parish Register*, lodged in the Genealogical Society Library.

569. Rev. L. T. Berguer (Ed.), *The British Essayists*, XXVIII (1823), p. 116.

570. Quoted in Abraham, *op. cit.*, p. 186, fn. 1.

571. Haygarth, *A Sketch, op. cit.*, pp. 75, 76.

572. *The Gentleman's Magazine*, 52 (1782), p. 473.

573. J. Howlett, *An Examination of Dr Price's Essay on the Population of England and Wales* (Maidstone, 1781), p. 83, fn.

574. *Ibid*, p. 94.

575. Howlett, *Observations, op. cit.*, p. 8.

576. Howlett, *An Examination, op. cit.*, p. 94.

577. A. Young (Ed.), *Annals of Agriculture*, VII (1786), p. 455.

578. J. Plymley, *General View of the Agriculture of Shropshire* (1803), pp. 343, 344.
579. J. Holt, *General View of the Agriculture of the County of Lancaster* (1795), p. 208, fn. 2.
580. Heysham, *op. cit.*, pp. 668-75.
581. *The Gentleman's Magazine*, 66, 1 (1796), p. 112.
582. *Ibid*, 73, 1 (1803), p. 213.
583. *Ibid*, pp. 301, 302.
584. Hollingsworth, *op. cit.*, pp. 29-31.
585. *Ibid*, p. 46.
586. Phadke, *op. cit.*, p. 803.
587. Creighton, *op. cit.*, p. 624.
588. Creighton, *op. cit.*, p. 614; B. R. Mitchell and P. Deane, *Abstract of British Historical Statistics* (1962), p. 29.
589. *Royal Commission on Vaccination*, 1st Report (1889), p. 114.
590. See the "Irish Census 1841", *Parl. Pap. 1843/24*, p. 459, and "Tables of Deaths, Summary".
591. *The Epidemiological Society Report* (1852-53), p. 29.
592. "Irish Census 1841", *op. cit.*, pp. 434, 436, and "Tables of Deaths, Summary".
593. *Ibid*, "Tables of Deaths, Summary".
594. This is using Petty's population figure of 55,000 for Dublin; undoubtedly this is an underestimate, but some deaths were not registered so that the two under-enumerations appear to cancel each other out, giving a death rate of about 40 per 1000, a not unreasonable figure for a city the size of Dublin during this period. The decline of smallpox mortality in Dublin is indicated by the comparison of 1661-1745 when about twenty per cent of all deaths were due to smallpox with 1831-40 when it accounted for under three per cent of them.
595. See *Royal Commission on Vaccination*, 1st Report (1889), pp. 74, 215, 6th Report (1896), pp. 717, 718, 720; Edwardes, *op. cit.*, p. 55.

184

Note of Thanks

Much of the historical material covered in this book was gathered for my doctoral thesis, and I would like to thank Nuffield College for the research studentship which made this possible. Invaluable help and support was given by Professor Habakkuk who supervised the thesis, and Dr Max Hartwell who acted both as college tutor and devil's advocate for an opposing nutritional hypothesis. Dr Eric Jones cannot realise how important his interest in the work was to its completion, and his wit and humour, alongside numerous references garnered during his own research, are deeply appreciated. A number of other people supplied references and critical points which have been incorporated into the book, but I must single out Professor Keith Dumbell, who through a series of highly informative and stimulating discussions, has provided me with an indispensable virological sounding board. (It should be made clear however that he does not agree with every aspect of my analysis of the medical evidence.) Most of the medical side of the book was carried out during a one-year fellowship at the Wellcome Institute for the History of Medicine, and I must thank the Wellcome Trust for its financial help and Dr Edwin Clarke for his personal support during this period. The acting head of the Department of Sociology at Bedford College— Dr Ivor Burton—made the one-year fellowship possible by arranging my release from teaching duties, and the co-operation of the college in this is much appreciated. And finally I must thank Professor David Eversley for having puzzled me about population increase during the Industrial Revolution period, when he lectured to me as an undergraduate at Birmingham University; I hope this book will go some way towards answering a question so stimulatingly raised on that occasion.

NAME AND PLACE INDEX